Unveil
The Toxic Foods
Igniting your Inflammation

Karen J. Toups

TABLE OF CONTENT

INTRODUCTION

Roughly 60% of the US population deals with chronic inflammation. Many contemporary diseases, including diabetes, heart disease, autoimmune disorders, and even certain cancers, have this unseen enemy at their core. The rising prevalence of chronic illnesses in our culture begs the question: what is igniting this inflammatory fire?

It turns out that the food we eat frequently contains the solution. Perhaps the culprits behind our bodies' continual state of alert are the meals we eat every day, which are advertised as palatable and easy. The nutritious food our forefathers ate has been drastically altered by today's manufactured foods, which are full of hidden sugars and artificial chemicals. We have set the stage for inflammation to take root with our combination of inactive lifestyles, chronic stress, and poor dietary choices.

Inflammation and nutrition are two topics I never thought I'd have to become an authority in. It was in a pediatric hospital, watching in despair as my small daughter fought an enigmatic disease that physicians couldn't explain, rather than in a classroom or lab, that my quest started. I searched medical journals incessantly, trying to find solutions every night. It was during this frenzied quest that I came onto the expanding corpus of data connecting nutrition to inflammation and chronic illness.

That finding altered everything. Armed with this information, I altered our family's diet, removing suspected trigger foods and embracing anti-inflammatory alternatives. The turnaround in my daughter's health was nothing short of amazing. Her symptoms started to lessen, her vitality returned, and the sparkle came back to her eyes.

Witnessing this miraculous turnaround kindled a desire inside me. I couldn't help but worry how many others were suffering unnecessarily, uninformed of the healing power of food. I dived deeply into the field of nutritional research, aiming to learn the truth about inflammation and share it with as many people as possible.

Are you ready to quench the fires of inflammation and restore your vitality?

PART 1: THE FOUNDATION OF HEALING

Inflammation is a normal and necessary component of the body's healing process. When you get a cut, bruise, or infection, your immune system reacts by sending white blood cells to the damaged region to combat dangerous intruders and begin the healing process. Acute inflammation is a temporary reaction that typically lasts a few days.

However, not all inflammation is good. Chronic inflammation is an ongoing inflammatory reaction that may last months or even years. Chronic inflammation, as opposed to acute inflammation, which promotes healing, may harm healthy tissues and organs. This sort of inflammation is typically overlooked, giving it the label "the silent saboteur."

What causes chronic inflammation?

Chronic inflammation may be caused by many reasons, including:

1. Infections: Persistent infections that the body cannot completely eradicate might cause chronic inflammation.
2. Autoimmune Disorders**: In conditions such as rheumatoid arthritis and lupus, the immune system erroneously attacks healthy tissues, resulting in persistent inflammation.
3. Environmental Factors**: Prolonged exposure to pollution, industrial chemicals, and other poisons may lead to chronic inflammation.
4. Lifestyle Factors: Poor nutrition, lack of exercise, smoking, and chronic stress are all major contributors to chronic inflammation.

Signs Your Body is Fighting Inflammation

Chronic inflammation often advances quietly, but there are certain indicators that your body may be struggling with it:

- Persistent Fatigue: Feeling exhausted even after a full night's sleep.
- Joint and Muscle Pain: Unexplained aches and pains in your joints or muscles.
- Digestive Issues: Conditions such as constipation, diarrhea, or acid reflux.
- Mental Health Issues: Chronic inflammation has been related to conditions including depression and anxiety.
- Weight Change: Unexplained weight loss or increase.

- Frequent Infections: Experiencing sickness more often than normal.

If you believe that you have persistent inflammation, you should see a doctor. They may prescribe blood tests to look for inflammatory markers like CRP or ESR.

Inflammation and Major Diseases

Chronic inflammation has been related to numerous major illnesses, making it an important area of concern for general health.

1. Heart Disease: Inflammation may damage the lining of the arteries, resulting in atherosclerosis (artery hardening), which is a substantial risk factor for heart attacks and strokes.
2. Type 2 Diabetes: Chronic inflammation may disrupt insulin signaling, resulting in insulin resistance and ultimately type 2 diabetes.
3. Cancer: Inflammatory processes may increase the development and spread of cancer cells.
4. Alzheimer's disease: It is thought that inflammation in the brain contributes to the development of Alzheimer's disease.
5. Autoimmune Diseases: Chronic inflammation directly causes conditions such as rheumatoid arthritis and lupus.

The Healing Potential of an Anti-Inflammatory Diet

An anti-inflammatory diet is intended to minimize chronic inflammation in the body, which may help prevent and manage a variety of health issues. This diet focuses on eating foods that are anti-inflammatory while avoiding those that might cause inflammation. The idea is to help the body's natural healing processes and improve overall health.

Foods that promote healing

Certain foods are known to have anti-inflammatory effects and may be useful friends in the battle against chronic inflammation. Here are some crucial things to include into your diet:

1. Fruits and Vegetables: These are high in antioxidants, vitamins, and minerals, which assist to reduce inflammation. Berries, leafy greens, tomatoes, and cruciferous vegetables like broccoli and cauliflower are especially useful.
2. Healthy Fats: Omega-3 fatty acids found in fatty fish (such as salmon and mackerel), flaxseeds, chia seeds, and walnuts have powerful anti-inflammatory properties
3. Whole Grains: Whole grains, such as brown rice, quinoa, and oats, retain fiber and minerals, potentially reducing inflammation

4. Nuts and Seeds: Almonds, walnuts, flaxseeds, and chia seeds are high in healthful fats and antioxidants.
5. Herbs and Spices: Turmeric, ginger, garlic, and cinnamon have significant anti-inflammatory effects and may be readily included into meals
6. Green Tea: Green tea is high in antioxidants and can help decrease inflammation and improve general health.

Inflammatory Foods to Avoid:

Some foods may help decrease inflammation, while others might cause or exacerbate it. Here are some items that should be avoided or limited:

- Processed Foods: They often include harmful fats, sugars, and additives that may cause inflammation. Examples include fast meals, packaged snacks, and sugary cereals.
- Refined Carbohydrates: White bread, croissants, and other refined carbohydrates may raise blood sugar levels and promote inflammation.
- Sugary Beverages: Sodas, energy drinks, and other sugary beverages may cause inflammation and lead to a variety of health problems.
- Red and Processed Meats: Excessive intake of red meat and processed meats, such as sausages and bacon, has been related to inflammation.
- Trans Fats: Trans fats, found in many fried meals, baked products, and margarine, are known to cause inflammation.
- Excessive Alcohol: While moderate alcohol intake has certain health advantages, excessive drinking may cause inflammation and other health issues.

The Function of Whole Foods in Reducing Inflammation

Whole foods are little processed and maintain their original nutrients, making them a crucial component of any anti-inflammatory diet. This is how they help:

1. Nutrient Density: Whole foods provide vitamins, minerals, and antioxidants that boost the immune system and decrease inflammation.
2. Fiber Content: High-fiber meals, such as fruits, vegetables, and whole grains, assist to maintain a healthy gut flora, which is important for inflammation regulation.
3. Healthy Fats: Whole foods such as nuts, seeds, and avocados include healthy fats that may lower inflammation and improve heart health.
4. Natural components: Many whole foods include natural anti-inflammatory components, including polyphenols in fruits and vegetables and omega-3 fatty acids in fish and flaxseeds.

Water, Nature's Ultimate Healer

Water is often considered to be the essence of life, and for good reason. It accounts for about 60% of the human body and is involved in practically all biological functions. Water is essential for preserving health and well-being, since it regulates body temperature and aids in digestion. It has several therapeutic effects, making it one of the most essential components for life.

The Importance of Hydration in Detoxification

Hydration is essential for the body's detoxification processes. Here's how keeping hydrated may help your body cleanse.

1. Kidney Function: The kidneys filter waste from the blood and excrete it as urine. Adequate water consumption ensures that the kidneys work properly, reducing the accumulation of toxins.
2. Liver Function: The liver plays a crucial function in detoxifying by breaking down toxic chemicals. Water improves liver function by flushing out toxins more effectively
3. Additionally, water supports digestion by breaking down food and absorbing minerals. It prevents constipation by lubricating the digestive tract
4. Skin Health: Proper hydration is vital for healthy skin. Water flushes away impurities via perspiration and keeps the skin moisturized, lowering the risk of skin problems
5. Cellular Health: Water is essential for the healthy operation of all cells in the body. Hydration promotes effective food delivery and waste removal in cells.

How Water Removes Inflammation from the Body

Water may help regulate and relieve inflammation in a variety of ways.

- Hydration and Inflammation: Staying hydrated helps keep body fluids in balance, which is essential for lowering inflammation. Dehydration may worsen inflammatory diseases by making it difficult for the body to eliminate toxins.
- Joint Health: Water lubricates joints, minimizing friction and inflammation. Proper hydration may ease symptoms of inflammatory illnesses such as arthritis. It also promotes blood circulation, delivering oxygen and nutrients to inflamed tissues and removing waste materials.
- Water helps speed up healing and decrease inflammation. It also assists in detoxification by flushing away toxins via the kidneys and liver. Lowering the toxic burden in the body may assist to reduce inflammation.
- Immune Function: Hydration helps the immune system by producing lymph, a fluid that transports white blood cells and other immune cells throughout the body. A well-hydrated immune system is better able to combat infections and reduce inflammation.

To summarize, water is more than just a fundamental requirement; it is a potent healer that supports a variety of biological processes and aids in inflammation management. Staying hydrated helps your body's natural detoxification processes, supports joint health, improves circulation, and boosts your immune system. To fully realize the therapeutic power of water, drink lots of it every day.

PART 2: THE PATH TO SELF HEALING

Detoxification: Cleansing for Best Health

Detoxification is the process by which the body removes toxic chemicals to maintain maximum health and well-being. This natural process includes numerous organs, including the liver, kidneys, and skin, which collaborate to filter and eliminate pollutants. By supporting these organs via healthy habits, you may improve your body's detoxification and balance.

1. Liver Detoxification: The liver is the body's principal detox organ, digesting and neutralizing toxins before excreting them as water-soluble compounds.
   - Eat a nutrient-dense diet high in antioxidants, vitamins, and minerals to promote liver health. Berries, leafy greens, and herbs like parsley are very healthy. Herbal medicines such as milk thistle and dandelion root may improve liver function and detoxification.

2. Kidney Detoxification: The kidneys filter blood and eliminate waste and excess fluids via urine. They help maintain fluid and electrolyte balance.
   - Adequate hydration is critical for renal function. Drinking enough water helps the kidneys clear out impurities and avoid kidney stones. Consuming foods high in antioxidants and minerals, such cranberries and blueberries, may improve kidney function.

3. Skin Detoxification: Sweating eliminates toxins from the skin, the body's biggest organ. It functions as both a barrier and a detoxifying organ.
   - Regular exercise and sweat-inducing activities, including saunas, may help the skin clear pollutants. Keeping the skin clean and moisturized helps preserve its detoxifying functions.

Natural Detox Treatments: Herbs, Baths, and Teas

1. Herbs:
   - Milk Thistle: Milk thistle has liver-protective qualities and promotes liver cell regeneration and detoxification.
   - Dandelion Root: This herb enhances liver health and helps eliminate toxins.
   - Turmeric: Its anti-inflammatory and antioxidant qualities promote liver function and detoxification.

2. Detox Baths:
- Epsom Salt Bath: Epsom salt baths may remove toxins from the skin and offer magnesium, which helps muscular and nerve function.
- Baking Soda Bath: Baking soda may neutralize pollutants and soothe sensitive skin.

3. Detox Teas:
- Green Tea: High in antioxidants, it improves liver function and reduces inflammation.
- Ginger Tea: Ginger tea promotes digestion and contains anti-inflammatory effects that assist in detoxifying.
- Dandelion Tea: Promotes liver health and detoxification.

Fasting and Juicing for Anti-Inflammatory Properties

1. Fasting:
- Intermittent Fasting: A cycle of eating and fasting. It may decrease inflammation, enhance insulin sensitivity, and aid in detoxification.
- Benefits: Fasting rests the digestive system, enabling it to heal and cleanse. It may also increase autophagy, a process in which the body removes damaged cells and regenerates new ones.

2. Juicing: Juicing contains concentrated vitamins, minerals, and antioxidants that promote detoxification and decrease inflammation.
- Green Juice: Combine kale, spinach, cucumber, celery, green apple, and lemon to make a nutrient-dense drink.
- Beet juice: Blend beets, carrots, ginger, and oranges to make a cleansing and anti-inflammatory juice.

Gut Health: Where Healing Starts

The gut, sometimes known as the "second brain," plays an important role in general health. It is home to billions of bacteria, known as the gut microbiome, which are required for digestion, immunological function, and even mental wellness. Maintaining a healthy gut is essential for healing and well-being.

Gut inflammation may be induced by a variety of things, including a poor diet, stress, infections, and certain drugs. When the stomach becomes inflamed, it may cause a variety of health problems, including digestive disorders and systemic illnesses. Here's how inflammation affects gut health:

1. Immune Response: The gut houses a large part of the body's immune system. Inflammation in the gut may cause chronic inflammation throughout the body.

2. Additionally, the gut lining serves as a barrier to prevent hazardous chemicals from entering the circulation. Inflammation may compromise this barrier, resulting in a condition known as "leaky gut," where toxins and germs leak into the circulation, causing more inflammation.
3. Microbiota Imbalance: Maintaining a healthy gut microbiota helps reduce inflammation. Dysbiosis, or an imbalance in gut flora, may cause inflammation and lead to a variety of health conditions.

Rebuilding the Gut with Probiotics and Fermented Foods

Probiotics and fermented foods are effective ways to restore gut health. They bring good bacteria into the stomach, therefore balancing the microbiome and reducing inflammation.

1. Probiotics: Probiotics are living microorganisms that give health advantages when ingested in sufficient amounts
   - Probiotic supplements are available, although it is frequently preferable to get probiotics from natural dietary sources. Probiotics are abundant in yogurt, kefir, and some cheeses.
   - Probiotics may balance gut flora, improve digestion, enhance immunity, and decrease inflammation.

2. Fermented Foods: Fermented foods are those that have been through a process of lacto-fermentation, where natural bacteria feed on the sugar and starch in the food, creating beneficial enzymes, B vitamins, omega-3 fatty acids, and probiotics. Examples: Sauerkraut, kimchi, miso, tempeh, and kombucha are excellent sources of probiotics. Regular consumption of fermented foods can enhance gut health, improve digestion,

Natural Treatments for Gut Inflammation and Leaky Gut

Addressing gut inflammation and repairing a leaky gut requires a mix of dietary adjustments, lifestyle changes, and natural therapies.

1. Dietary Changes:
   - Anti-Inflammatory Diet: Consume complete, unprocessed foods high in antioxidants and anti-inflammatory properties. Include a variety of fruits, vegetables, whole grains, lean meats, and healthy fats. To reduce inflammation, avoid foods such refined sweets, processed meals, alcohol, and high-fat foods ([1]).

2. Lifestyle Modifications:
   - Stress Management: Chronic stress might lead to increased intestinal inflammation. Meditation, yoga, and deep breathing techniques may effectively control stress levels.
   - Regular Exercise: Physical exercise improves digestion and reduces inflammation.

3. Natural Remedies:
- Herbal Supplements: Turmeric, ginger, and licorice root are anti-inflammatory herbs that help improve gut health.
- Bone Broth: High in collagen and amino acids, bone broth helps promote intestinal healing and decrease inflammation.
- Aloe Vera: With its calming characteristics, aloe vera helps decrease stomach inflammation and improve healing.

Boosting Immunity for Inflammation Control

A healthy immune system is vital for reducing inflammation and improving overall health. The immune system is a complex network of cells, tissues, and organs that work together to protect the body against outside invaders such as bacteria, viruses, and poisons. Boosting your immunity may help your body handle inflammation more efficiently and promote recovery.

The immune system is essential for healing because it recognizes and eliminates dangerous chemicals while also mending damaged tissues. This is how it works.

1. Innate Immunity: This is the body's primary defense against infections. It comprises physical barriers like the skin and mucous membranes, as well as immune cells that fight intruders right away. Inflammation plays an important role in this response, helping to separate and remove dangerous molecules.
2. Adaptive Immunity: This system learns to detect certain infections and stores them for future encounters. The process includes producing antibodies and activating specialist immune cells. Adaptive immunity is necessary for long-term protection and allows the body to adapt more effectively to recurrent illnesses.
3. Inflammatory Control: While inflammation is a normal aspect of the immune system, persistent inflammation may be damaging. The immune system regulates inflammation, activating it when essential and suppressing it when not needed.

Boosting Immunity with Nutrition and Lifestyle

Boosting your immune system entails developing healthy behaviors that help it work. Here are a few major strategies:

1. Nutrition:
- Fruits and Vegetables: These provide vitamins, minerals, and antioxidants that boost immune function. Citrus fruits, strawberries, and bell peppers contain vitamin C, which is very beneficial for immunological health.
- Healthy Fats: Omega-3 fatty acids found in fatty fish, flaxseeds, and walnuts promote immune function and reduce inflammation.

- Protein: Enough protein is required for the formation of immune cells. Consume lean meats, chicken, fish, beans, and legumes.
- Probiotics: Yogurt, kefir, and fermented vegetables contain helpful bacteria that promote gut health and enhance the immune system.

2. Lifestyle:
- Regular Exercise: Physical exercise improves circulation and allows immune cells to travel freely throughout the body. Aim for 30 minutes of moderate activity on most days of the week.
- Adequate Sleep: Sleep is essential for immunological function. Aim for 7-9 hours of excellent sleep every night to aid in body repair and regeneration.
- Stress Management: Prolonged stress may deplete the immune system. Meditation, deep breathing techniques, and yoga may effectively control stress levels.
- Hydration: Staying hydrated benefits all physical systems, especially the immune system. Drink plenty of water throughout the day.

3. Avoiding Harmful Habits:
- Smoking: It lowers the immune system and raises the risk of illnesses. Quitting smoking may greatly enhance immunological function.
- Excessive Alcohol: Consuming too much alcohol might weaken the immune system. Limit your alcohol consumption to modest levels.

PART 3: FOODS THAT HEAL

Anti-inflammatory Pantry: What to Stock

Stocking your cupboard with anti-inflammatory foods is an excellent strategy to improve your health and lower chronic inflammation. Here are some key goods to have on hand:

1. Extra-Virgin Olive Oil: High in monounsaturated fats and polyphenols, it regulates immune responses and reduces inflammation.
2. Turmeric: Curcumin, the active ingredient in turmeric, is a powerful antioxidant that lowers inflammation markers.
3. Canned Tuna is a convenient source of omega-3 fatty acids, which are known for their anti-inflammatory properties.
4. Kidney Beans: Packed with dietary fiber, kidney beans promote a healthy gut microbiome and lower systemic inflammation.
5. Almonds: These nuts are rich in healthy fats, fiber, and antioxidants, making them a great anti-inflammatory snack.
6. Canned Tomatoes: High in lycopene, an antioxidant

Must-Have Foods to Reduce Inflammation

In addition to cupboard basics, include fresh items in your diet may also help decrease inflammation:

1. Fruits and Vegetables: Berries, leafy greens, tomatoes, and cruciferous vegetables like broccoli and cauliflower provide antioxidants and vitamins that fight inflammation.
2. Fatty Fish: Salmon, mackerel, and sardines are rich in omega-3 fatty acids.
3. Whole Grains: Brown rice, quinoa, and oats retain fiber and minerals to lower inflammation.
4. Nuts and Seeds: Walnuts, flaxseeds, and chia seeds provide beneficial lipids and antioxidants.
5. Herbs and Spices: Turmeric, ginger, garlic, and cinnamon have strong anti-inflammatory effects.

Making Balanced, Healing Meals using Natural Ingredients

Creating balanced meals with natural components will help you get the anti-inflammatory effects of these foods. Here are a few tips:

1. Begin with a Base of veggies: Fill half of your plate with a variety of colorful veggies. They provide important minerals and antioxidants.
2. Incorporate Lean Proteins: Include sources of lean protein such as fish, poultry, beans, or tofu. These assist to heal tissues and maintain immunological function.
3. Incorporate Whole Grains: Include one serving of whole grains, such as brown rice, quinoa, or whole wheat pasta. They include fiber and help keep blood sugar levels constant.
4. Include Healthy Fats: Cook with olive oil and add nuts or seeds to your meals to get your daily dosage of healthy fats.
5. Season with Herbs and Spices: Add taste and anti-inflammatory benefits to your meals using herbs and spices such as turmeric, ginger, and garlic.

The Healing Power of Herbs and Spices

Herbs and spices provide not just taste but also potent anti-inflammatory properties. Here are the three most effective:

1. Turmeric:
   - Benefits: Curcumin, the active ingredient in turmeric, has powerful anti-inflammatory and antioxidant capabilities. It helps alleviate inflammation and discomfort, particularly in illnesses such as arthritis. Add turmeric to curries, soups, and smoothies. Combine it with black pepper to increase absorption.

2. Ginger:
   - Benefits: Ginger includes gingerol, which has strong anti-inflammatory and antioxidant properties. It may help relieve muscular discomfort, stiffness, and inflammation in the intestines. Use fresh ginger in drinks, stir-fries, and smoothies. Ground ginger may be included into baked items and spice combinations.

3. Cinnamon:
   - Benefits: Cinnamon contains antioxidants and anti-inflammatory qualities. It may help decrease blood sugar levels and inflammation in the body. Add cinnamon to cereal, yogurt, and fruit. It may also be utilized in baked goods and savory recipes.

BREAKFAST AND BRUNCH

Berry-Kefir Smoothie

(per serving):

Calories: 200

Fat: 7g

Protein: 8g

Carbs: 30g

Fiber: 8g

Sugars: 14g

Prep Time: 5 minutes Serving Size: 1 smoothie (about 16 ounces)

1 cup mixed berries

1/2 cup plain kefir

1/2 cup unsweetened almond milk

1 tablespoon chia seeds

1/2 tablespoon honey or maple syrup (optional)

1/2 teaspoon ground turmeric

1/4 teaspoon ground cinnamon

1/4 teaspoon ground ginger

A handful of spinach

Thoroughly wash the berries. Thawing frozen berries is not necessary if utilizing them.

Fill a blender with the following ingredients: spinach, berries, kefir, almond milk, chia seeds, honey, maple syrup, turmeric, cinnamon, ginger, and ginger.

Process the ingredients on high until it becomes creamy and smooth. To get the right consistency, thin down any extra smoothie by adding a little amount of almond milk.

Transfer to a glass.

Turmeric Latte

(per serving):

Calories: 120 kcal

Fat: 8g

Protein: 1g

Carbs: 11g

Fiber: 1g

Sugars: 7g

Prep Time: 5 minutes Cooking Time: 5 minutes Total Time: 10 minutes
Serving Size: 1 cup (about 8 ounces)

1 cup unsweetened almond milk

1/2 teaspoon ground turmeric

1/4 teaspoon ground cinnamon

1/4 teaspoon ground ginger

A pinch of black pepper

1 teaspoon coconut oil or ghee

1 teaspoon honey or maple syrup

Warm, but not boiling, almond milk should be heated in a small saucepan over medium heat.

Incorporate the ginger, cinnamon, turmeric, and black pepper into the heated milk. Stirring constantly will help avoid clumping.

If using, stir in the ghee or coconut oil and honey or maple syrup until well mixed.

To let the flavors to merge, lower the heat to low and simmer the mixture for three to five minutes.

You may give the latte a brief blender run to get a frother texture.

Warm up the turmeric latte by pouring it into a cup.

Mango-Kale Smoothie

((per serving):

Calories: 190

Fat: 5g

Protein: 3g

Carbs: 37g

Fiber: 7g

Sugars: 25g

Prep Time: 5 minutes Serving Size: 1 smoothie (about 16 ounces)

1 cup fresh or frozen mango chunks

1/2 cup chopped kale (remove tough stems)

1/2 banana

1/2 cup unsweetened almond milk

1/2 cup water or coconut water

1 tablespoon chia seeds

1/2 teaspoon ground turmeric

1/2 teaspoon grated ginger

A squeeze of fresh lime juice (optional, for a tangy twist)

If using fresh mango, peel and chop into chunks. Wash and chop the kale, removing the tough stems.

Add all the ingredients (mango, kale, banana, almond milk, water or coconut water, chia seeds, turmeric, ginger, and lime juice) to a blender.

Blend on high until the mixture is smooth and creamy. Add more water if needed to reach your desired consistency.

Cherry-Mocha Smoothie

(per serving):

Calories: 200

Prep Time: 5 minutes Serving Size: 1 smoothie (about 16 ounces)

Fat: 9g

Protein: 5g

1 cup frozen cherries

1/2 tablespoon maple syrup

carbs: 29g

1/2 cup unsweetened almond milk

1/2 teaspoon vanilla extract

Fiber: 6g

1/2 cup brewed coffee, cooled

1/2 small beetroot, cooked and peeled

Sugars: 17g

1 tablespoon unsweetened cocoa powder

1 tablespoon almond butter

If using raw beetroot, cook and peel it beforehand

Add all the ingredients (frozen cherries, almond milk, coffee, cocoa powder, almond butter, maple syrup, vanilla extract, and beetroot) to a blender.

Blend on high until the mixture is smooth and creamy. If the smoothie is too thick, add a bit more almond milk or coffee to reach your desired consistency.

Golden Milk

(per serving):

Calories: 130

Fat: 9g

Protein: 1g

Carbohydrates: 12g

Fiber: 1g

Sugars: 7g

Prep Time: 5 minutes Cooking Time: 5 minutes Total Time: 10 minutes
Serving Size: 1 cup (about 8 ounces)

1 cup unsweetened coconut milk

1/2 teaspoon ground turmeric

1/4 teaspoon ground cinnamon

1/4 teaspoon ground ginger

A pinch of black pepper

1/2 teaspoon vanilla extract (optional)

1 teaspoon coconut oil

1 teaspoon maple syrup or honey

Chop the fresh pineapple into bite-sized pieces if using it.

Put the cottage cheese and pineapple pieces in a bowl. Gently stir to combine.

Garnish with chia seeds, drizzle with honey, and, if you'd like, a dash of cinnamon.

Eat right now, or chill if making ahead.

Avocado-Banana Smoothie

((per serving):

Calories: 280

Fat: 14g

Protein: 4g

Carbs: 38g

Fiber: 9g

Sugars: 17g

Prep Time: 5 minutes Serving Size: 1 smoothie (about 16 ounces)

1/2 ripe avocado

1 ripe banana

1 cup unsweetened almond milk

1 tablespoon chia seeds

1/2 tablespoon honey or maple syrup (optional)

1/2 teaspoon ground turmeric

1/4 teaspoon ground cinnamon

1/4 teaspoon ground ginger

A handful of spinach

Scoop out the flesh of the avocado and peel the banana.

Add the avocado, banana, almond milk, chia seeds, honey/maple syrup, turmeric, cinnamon, ginger, and spinach (if using) to a blender.

Blend on high until the mixture is smooth and creamy. If the smoothie is too thick, add a little more almond milk to reach your desired consistency.

Avocado & Kale Omelet

(per serving):

Calories: 300

Fat: 24g

Protein: 12g

Carbs: 10g

Fiber: 6g

Sugars: 2g

Prep Time: 10 minutes Cooking Time: 10 minutes Total Time: 20 minutes
Serving Size: 1 omelet (about 2 eggs)

2 large eggs

1/2 avocado, sliced

1/2 cup fresh kale, chopped

1 tablespoon olive oil or coconut oil

1/4 teaspoon garlic powder

1/4 teaspoon onion powder

Salt and pepper to taste

Wash and chop the kale. Slice the avocado.

In a non-stick skillet, heat the olive oil or coconut oil over medium heat.

Add the chopped kale to the skillet and cook for about 2-3 minutes, or until wilted and slightly crispy.

In a bowl, beat the eggs with garlic powder, onion powder, salt, and pepper.

Pour the beaten eggs into the skillet over the kale. Let the eggs cook undisturbed for about 2-3 minutes, or until the edges start to set.

Carefully place the avocado slices on one half of the omelet.

Once the omelet is mostly set, fold it in half over the avocado. Cook for another 1-2 minutes until the eggs are fully set.

Slide the omelet onto a plate and enjoy it warm.

Egg Salad Avocado Toast

(per serving):

Calories: 350

Fat: 22g

Protein: 14g

Carbs: 30g

Fiber: 8g

Sugars: 4g

Prep Time: 10 minutes Cooking Time: 10 minutes Total Time: 20 minutes
Serving Size: 1 slice of toast with egg salad

For the Egg Salad:

4 large eggs

2 tablespoons avocado mayonnaise or regular mayonnaise if preferred

1 tablespoon Dijon mustard

1 tablespoon chopped fresh dill or 1 teaspoon dried dill

1 tablespoon chopped chives or green onions

Salt and pepper to taste

For the Toast:

1 slice of whole grain bread

1 ripe avocado

A squeeze of lemon juice

Salt and pepper to taste

Cook the Eggs:

- Place the eggs in a saucepan and cover with water.

- Bring to a boil over medium-high heat, then cover and reduce heat to low. Simmer for 10 minutes.

- Remove the eggs and place them in an ice bath or under cold running water to cool. Once cool, peel and chop the eggs.

Prepare the Egg Salad:

- In a mixing bowl, combine the chopped eggs, avocado mayonnaise, Dijon mustard, dill, and chives. Mix well.

- Season with salt and pepper to taste.

Prepare the Toast:

- Toast the slice of bread to your desired level of crispness.

- While the bread is toasting, mash the avocado in a small bowl and mix in the lemon juice, salt, and pepper.

Assemble the Toast:

- Spread the mashed avocado evenly on the toasted bread.

- Top with a generous portion of egg salad.

- Garnish with additional chives or dill if desired.

Beetroot Smoothie

((per serving):

Calories: 180

Fat: 4g

Protein: 3g

Carbs: 36g

Fiber: 7g

Sugars: 20g

Prep Time: 10 minutes Serving Size: 1 smoothie (about 16 ounces)

1 small raw beetroot, peeled and chopped

1/2 cup frozen mixed berries

1/2 banana, sliced

1/2 cup unsweetened almond milk

1/4 cup orange juice, freshly squeezed if possible

1 tablespoon chia seeds

1/2 teaspoon ground ginger

1/2 teaspoon ground cinnamon

1/2 teaspoon turmeric powder

1 teaspoon honey or maple syrup

Peel and chop the beetroot. If you're using fresh berries, you might want to add a few ice cubes to make the smoothie cold.

Add the beetroot, mixed berries, banana, almond milk, orange juice, chia seeds, ginger, cinnamon, turmeric, and honey/maple syrup (if using) to a blender.

Blend on high until the mixture is smooth and creamy. If the smoothie is too thick, add a little more almond milk or orange juice to reach your desired consistency.

Pineapple-Ginger Smoothie

(per serving):

Calories: 150

Fat: 4g

Protein: 2g

Carbs: 30g

Fiber: 5g

Sugars: 18g

Prep Time: 5 minutes Serving Size: 1 smoothie (about 16 ounces)

1 cup fresh or frozen pineapple chunks

1/2 cup unsweetened coconut water or water

1/2 cup unsweetened almond milk

1 tablespoon fresh ginger, peeled and grated

1/2 banana

1 tablespoon chia seeds

1 teaspoon honey or maple syrup

A handful of spinach

If using fresh pineapple, peel, core, and chop it into chunks. Peel and grate the ginger.

Add the pineapple, coconut water, almond milk, ginger, banana (if using), chia seeds, and sweetener to a blender.

Blend on high until the mixture is smooth and creamy. If the smoothie is too thick, add a little more coconut water or almond milk to reach your desired consistency.

Blueberry-Spinach Smoothie

(per serving):

Calories: 220

Fat: 8g

Protein: 5g

Carbs: 30g

Fiber: 8g

Sugars: 17g

Prep Time: 5 minutes Serving Size: 1 smoothie (about 16 ounces)

1 cup fresh or frozen blueberries

1 cup fresh spinach

1/2 cup unsweetened almond milk

1/2 cup plain coconut yogurt

1 tablespoon chia seeds

1 teaspoon flax seeds (optional)

1/2 tablespoon maple syrup or honey

1/4 teaspoon ground turmeric

1/2 teaspoon vanilla extract

If using frozen blueberries, there is no need to thaw them. Wash the spinach if it's not pre-washed.

Add all the ingredients (blueberries, spinach, almond milk, coconut yogurt, chia seeds, flaxseeds, maple syrup/honey, turmeric, and vanilla extract) to a blender.

Blend on high until the mixture is smooth and creamy. If the smoothie is too thick, add a bit more almond milk to reach your desired consistency.

Spinach & Egg Scramble

((per serving):

Calories: 240

Fat: 18g

Protein: 14g

Carbs: 8g

Fiber: 2g

Sugars: 3g

Prep Time: 5 minutes Cooking Time: 10 minutes Total Time: 15 minutes
Serving Size: 1 serving

2 large eggs

1 cup fresh spinach, chopped

1/4 cup diced onion

1/4 cup diced bell pepper (any color)

1 tablespoon olive oil

Salt and pepper to taste

1/4 teaspoon ground turmeric

1 tablespoon nutritional yeast

Wash and chop the spinach. Dice the onion and bell pepper.

In a non-stick skillet, heat olive oil over medium heat.

Add the diced onion and bell pepper to the skillet. Sauté for about 3-4 minutes until they become soft.

Add the chopped spinach to the skillet and cook for an additional 1-2 minutes until wilted.

In a bowl, whisk the eggs with a pinch of salt, pepper, and ground turmeric (if using). Pour the egg mixture over the vegetables in the skillet.

Allow the eggs to cook undisturbed for about 1 minute, then gently stir and scramble until fully cooked, about 3-4 minutes.

If using, sprinkle the nutritional yeast over the scramble and stir to combine.

VEGETARIAN AND VEGAN

Caprese-Stuffed Portobello Mushrooms

(per serving):

Calories: 150

Fat: 10g

Protein: 7g

Carbs: 10g

Fiber: 2g

Sugars: 6g

Prep Time: 10 minutes Cooking Time: 20 minutes Total Time: 30 minutes
Serving Size: 1 mushroom cap (makes 4 servings)

4 large portobello mushroom caps

1 cup cherry tomatoes, halved

1 cup fresh basil leaves, chopped

1/2 cup mozzarella cheese, shredded

2 tablespoons extra virgin olive oil

1 tablespoon balsamic vinegar

1 clove garlic, minced

Salt and black pepper to taste

Preheat your oven to 375°F (190°C).

Clean the portobello mushroom caps with a damp paper towel. Remove the stems and scoop out the gills using a spoon.

In a mixing bowl, combine the cherry tomatoes, chopped basil, mozzarella cheese, minced garlic, olive oil, balsamic vinegar, salt, and black pepper.

Place the mushroom caps on a baking sheet lined with parchment paper. Spoon the tomato and cheese mixture into each mushroom cap, distributing it evenly.

Bake in the preheated oven for 20 minutes, or until the mushrooms are tender and the cheese is melted and bubbly.

Remove from the oven and let cool for a few minutes before serving.

Sweet Potato-Black Bean Tacos

(per serving, 2 tacos):

Calories: 350

Fat: 8g

Protein: 12g

Carbs: 56g

Fiber: 12g

Sugars: 10g

Prep Time: 15 minutes Cooking Time: 20 minutes Total Time: 35 minutes
Serving Size: 2 tacos (about 1 cup filling per taco)

1 large sweet potato, peeled and diced

1 tablespoon olive oil

1/2 teaspoon ground cumin

1/2 teaspoon paprika

1/4 teaspoon ground turmeric

1/4 teaspoon garlic powder

1/4 teaspoon onion powder

Salt and black pepper to taste

1 can (15 oz) black beans, drained and rinsed

1/2 cup diced red onion

1/2 cup diced bell pepper (any color)

1/4 cup chopped fresh cilantro

Juice of 1 lime

4 small corn or gluten-free tortillas

Avocado slices, salsa, shredded lettuce, chopped tomatoes

Preheat the oven to 400°F (200°C). Toss the diced sweet potato with olive oil, cumin, paprika, turmeric, garlic powder, onion powder, salt, and pepper. Spread evenly on a baking sheet.

Roast in the oven for 20 minutes or until tender and lightly browned, stirring halfway through.

In a bowl, combine black beans, diced red onion, diced bell pepper, cilantro, and lime juice. Season with salt and pepper to taste.

Heat the tortillas in a dry skillet over medium heat until warm and pliable, about 30 seconds per side.

Fill each tortilla with roasted sweet potatoes and black bean mixture. Top with optional toppings if desired.

Lentil and Spinach Stew

(per serving, 1 cup):

Calories: 180

Fat: 5g

Protein: 9g

Carbs: 27g

Fiber: 9g

Sugars: 6g

Prep Time: 10 minutes Cooking Time: 30 minutes Total Time: 40 minutes
Serving Size: 1 cup (about 8 ounces)

1 tablespoon olive oil

1 medium onion, diced

3 garlic cloves, minced

1 large carrot, diced

1 celery stalk, diced

1 cup dried green or brown lentils, rinsed

1 can (14.5 ounces) diced tomatoes

4 cups vegetable broth

2 cups fresh spinach, chopped

1 teaspoon ground turmeric

1/2 teaspoon ground cumin

1/2 teaspoon smoked paprika

1/4 teaspoon ground black pepper

1/4 teaspoon sea salt

1 bay leaf (optional)

Heat olive oil in a large pot over medium heat. Add the onion, garlic, carrot, and celery. Cook for about 5-7 minutes, or until the vegetables are softened.

Stir in the turmeric, cumin, paprika, black pepper, and salt. Cook for another 1-2 minutes until fragrant.

Add the lentils, diced tomatoes, vegetable broth, and bay leaf (if using). Bring to a boil.

Reduce the heat to low and let the stew simmer for about 20-25 minutes, or until the lentils are tender.

Stir in the chopped spinach and cook for an additional 5 minutes, until the spinach is wilted and the stew is heated through.

Taste and adjust seasoning if needed. Remove the bay leaf before serving.

Vegetable Paella

((per serving):

Calories: 250

Fat: 7g

Protein: 7g

Carbohydrates: 40g

Fiber: 7g

Sugars: 8g

Prep Time: 15 minutes Cooking Time: 35 minutes Total Time: 50 minutes
Serving Size: 1 cup (about 200g)

1 tablespoon olive oil

1 onion, finely chopped

3 garlic cloves, minced

1 red bell pepper, chopped

1 yellow bell pepper, chopped

1 zucchini, sliced

1 cup cherry tomatoes, halved

1 cup green beans, trimmed and cut into pieces

1 cup peas (fresh or frozen)

1 1/2 cups short-grain brown rice

1/4 teaspoon saffron threads or 1/2 teaspoon turmeric as a substitute

1 teaspoon smoked paprika

1/2 teaspoon ground cumin

1/4 teaspoon ground black pepper

1/4 teaspoon cayenne pepper (optional, for heat)

3 cups vegetable broth

1 lemon, cut into wedges

Fresh parsley, chopped

Heat the olive oil in a large skillet or paella pan over medium heat. Add the onion and garlic and cook until softened, about 5 minutes.

Stir in the red and yellow bell peppers and zucchini. Cook for another 5 minutes, until vegetables begin to soften.

Add the saffron (or turmeric), smoked paprika, cumin, black pepper, and cayenne pepper (if using). Stir to coat the vegetables in the spices.

Stir in the rice, making sure it is well-coated with the spices. Pour in the vegetable broth and bring to a boil.

Reduce heat to low, cover, and simmer for about 20 minutes.

After 20 minutes, add the cherry tomatoes, green beans, and peas. Stir gently, cover, and cook for another 10 minutes, or until the rice is tender and the liquid has been absorbed.

Remove from heat and let the paella sit, covered, for 5 minutes.

Garnish with chopped parsley and serve with lemon wedges.

Mushroom Risotto

(per serving):

Calories: 250

Fat: 8g

Protein: 5g

Carbs: 40g

Fiber: 2g

Sugars: 4g

Prep Time: 10 minutes Cooking Time: 30 minutes Total Time: 40 minutes
Serving Size: 1 cup

1 cup Arborio rice

1 tablespoon olive oil

1 medium onion, finely chopped

2 cloves garlic, minced

2 cups mushrooms, sliced such as cremini or shiitake

1/4 cup white wine (optional)

4 cups vegetable broth

1/4 cup nutritional yeast

2 tablespoons fresh parsley, chopped

Salt and pepper to taste

Heat the vegetable broth in a saucepan and keep it warm on low heat.

In a large skillet, heat the olive oil over medium heat. Add the chopped onion and cook until translucent, about 5 minutes. Add the garlic and mushrooms and cook until the mushrooms are softened, about 5 minutes.

Stir in the Arborio rice and cook for 1-2 minutes until lightly toasted.

If using white wine, add it now and cook until the wine is mostly absorbed.

Begin adding the warm vegetable broth, one ladleful at a time, stirring frequently. Allow the liquid to be absorbed before adding more broth. Continue this process until the rice is creamy and cooked through, about 20-25 minutes.

Stir in the nutritional yeast, if using, and season with salt and pepper. Garnish with fresh parsley.

Chickpea and Spinach Curry

((per serving):

Calories: 250

Fat: 14g

Protein: 8g

Carbs: 28g

Fiber: 7g

Sugars: 6g

Prep Time: 10 minutes Cooking Time: 25 minutes Total Time: 35 minutes
Serving Size: 1 cup (about 8 ounces)

1 tablespoon olive oil

1 onion, finely chopped

3 garlic cloves, minced

1 tablespoon fresh ginger, minced

1 can (15 oz) chickpeas, drained and rinsed

1 can (15 oz) diced tomatoes

1 cup coconut milk

2 cups fresh spinach, chopped

1 tablespoon curry powder

1/2 teaspoon ground turmeric

1/2 teaspoon ground cumin

1/2 teaspoon ground coriander

1/4 teaspoon cayenne pepper

Salt and black pepper to taste

Fresh cilantro for garnish

In a large skillet or saucepan, heat the olive oil over medium heat.

Add the onion and cook until translucent, about 5 minutes. Add the garlic and ginger and cook for another 1-2 minutes.

Stir in the curry powder, turmeric, cumin, coriander, and cayenne pepper (if using). Cook for 1 minute to toast the spices.

Add the chickpeas and diced tomatoes to the skillet. Stir well to combine.

Pour in the coconut milk, bring the mixture to a simmer, and cook for 10 minutes, allowing the flavors to meld and the sauce to thicken slightly.

Stir in the chopped spinach and cook for an additional 5 minutes until the spinach is wilted.

Season with salt and black pepper to taste.

Garnish with fresh cilantro if desired and serve hot.

Vegan Buddha Bowl

(per serving):

Calories: 500

Fat: 22g

Protein: 14g

Carbs: 60g

Fiber: 12g

Sugars: 9g

Prep Time: 15 minutes Cooking Time: 20 minutes Total Time: 35 minutes
Serving Size: 1 bowl

For the Bowl:

1 cup cooked quinoa

1 cup roasted sweet potatoes (cubed)

1 cup steamed broccoli florets

1/2 cup shredded red cabbage

1/2 avocado, sliced

1/4 cup chickpeas (cooked or canned, rinsed)

2 tablespoons sesame seeds

For the Dressing:

2 tablespoons tahini

1 tablespoon lemon juice

1 tablespoon tamari (gluten-free soy sauce) or coconut aminos

1 teaspoon maple syrup

1 clove garlic, minced

Water, as needed to thin the dressing

Rinse quinoa under cold water. Cook according to package instructions (usually 1 part quinoa to 2 parts water, bring to a boil, then simmer for about 15 minutes). Let cool.

Preheat the oven to 400°F (200°C). Toss cubed sweet potatoes with a bit of olive oil, salt, and pepper. Spread on a baking sheet and roast for 20 minutes, or until tender.

Steam broccoli florets for about 5-7 minutes until tender but still crisp. Set aside.

In a small bowl, whisk together tahini, lemon juice, tamari or coconut aminos, maple syrup, and minced garlic. Add water a little at a time until the dressing reaches your desired consistency.

In a large bowl, arrange cooked quinoa, roasted sweet potatoes, steamed broccoli, shredded red cabbage, avocado slices, and chickpeas. Drizzle with tahini dressing and sprinkle with sesame seeds.

Vegan Lentil Soup

(per serving):

Calories: 180

Fat: 4g

Protein: 10g

Carbs: 28g

Fiber: 9g

Sugars: 6g

Prep Time: 10 minutes Cooking Time: 30 minutes Total Time: 40 minutes
Serving Size: 1 cup

1 tablespoon olive oil

1 medium onion, diced

2 cloves garlic, minced

2 medium carrots, diced

2 celery stalks, diced

1 cup dried green or brown lentils, rinsed and drained

1 can (14.5 ounces) diced tomatoes

6 cups vegetable broth

1 teaspoon ground cumin

1 teaspoon smoked paprika

1/2 teaspoon ground turmeric

1/2 teaspoon dried thyme

1 bay leaf

Salt and pepper to taste

2 cups spinach or kale, chopped

In a large pot, heat the olive oil over medium heat. Add the onion and garlic, and sauté until the onion is translucent, about 5 minutes.

Stir in the carrots and celery and cook for an additional 5 minutes.

Add the lentils, diced tomatoes, vegetable broth, cumin, paprika, turmeric, thyme, bay leaf, salt, and pepper. Bring to a boil.

Reduce heat and let the soup simmer for 25-30 minutes, or until the lentils and vegetables are tender.

If using spinach or kale, stir it in during the last 5 minutes of cooking.

Remove the bay leaf before serving. Adjust seasoning to taste

MEAT, POULTRY AND PROTEIN

Turmeric Chicken

(per serving, based on 4 servings total):

Calories: 250

Fat: 18g

Protein: 21g

Carbs: 2g

Fiber: 0.5g

Sugars: 0g

Prep Time: 15 minutes Cooking Time: 25 minutes Total Time: 40 minutes
Serving Size: 1 serving (about 4 ounces of chicken

4 boneless, skinless chicken thighs (about 1 pound)

2 tablespoons olive oil

2 teaspoons ground turmeric

1 teaspoon ground cumin

1 teaspoon paprika

1/2 teaspoon ground black pepper

1/2 teaspoon garlic powder

1/2 teaspoon onion powder

1/2 teaspoon salt or to taste

1 tablespoon lemon juice

1 tablespoon chopped fresh cilantro

Preheat your oven to 375°F (190°C).

Pat the chicken thighs dry with paper towels.

In a small bowl, mix the turmeric, cumin, paprika, black pepper, garlic powder, onion powder, and salt. Rub this spice mixture all over the chicken thighs.

Heat olive oil in an oven-proof skillet over medium-high heat. Add the chicken thighs and seat for 3-4 minutes on each side, until golden brown.

Transfer the skillet to the preheated oven and bake for 20-25 minutes, or until the chicken is fully cooked and reaches an internal temperature of 165°F (74°C).

Remove from the oven, drizzle with lemon juice, and garnish with chopped cilantro if desired.

Serve warm with your choice of side dishes.

Ginger-Garlic Chicken Stir-Fry

(per serving):

Calories: 250

Fat: 10g

Protein: 30g

Carbs: 15g

Fiber: 4g

Sugars: 6g

Prep Time: 15 minutes Cooking Time: 10 minutes Total Time: 25 minutes
Serving Size: 1 cup

1 lb (450g) chicken breast, thinly sliced

1 tablespoon olive oil

2 cloves garlic, minced

1 tablespoon fresh ginger, minced

1 red bell pepper, sliced

1 cup broccoli florets

1 medium carrot, julienned

2 tablespoons coconut aminos or gluten-free soy sauce

1 tablespoon rice vinegar

1 teaspoon sesame oil (optional)

1 tablespoon chopped fresh cilantro

Salt and pepper to taste

Slice the chicken breast and vegetables. Mince the garlic and ginger.

In a large skillet or wok, heat the olive oil over medium-high heat.

Add the sliced chicken to the skillet and cook for 5-7 minutes, or until the chicken is no longer pink and starts to brown.

Add the minced garlic and ginger to the skillet. Stir-fry for 1 minute until fragrant.

Add the bell pepper, broccoli, and carrot to the skillet. Stir-fry for another 5 minutes, or until the vegetables are tender-crisp.

Stir in the coconut aminos and rice vinegar. Cook for an additional 1-2 minutes, ensuring everything is well-coated and heated through.

Drizzle with sesame oil if using, and season with salt and pepper to taste.

Garnish with chopped cilantro if desired, and serve warm.

Lemon-Herb Roasted Chicken

((per serving, based on 4 servings):

Calories: 300

Fat: 16g

Protein: 35g

Carbs: 2g

Fiber: 0g

Sugars: 1g

Prep Time: 15 minutes Cooking Time: 1 hour 15 minutes Total Time: 1 hour 30 minutes Serving Size: 1 chicken breast (about 4 ounces)

1 whole chicken (about 4 pounds)	1 teaspoon paprika
2 tablespoons olive oil	1 teaspoon ground black pepper
1 lemon, cut into wedges	1 teaspoon sea salt
4 cloves garlic, minced	1 onion, quartered
2 tablespoons fresh rosemary, chopped or 2 teaspoons dried rosemary	1 cup low-sodium chicken broth
2 tablespoons fresh thyme, chopped or 2 teaspoons dried thyme	

Preheat your oven to 425°F (220°C).

Pat the chicken dry with paper towels. Rub the outside of the chicken with olive oil.

Sprinkle garlic, rosemary, thyme, paprika, black pepper, and sea salt all over the chicken, including inside the cavity. Place the lemon wedges and quartered onion inside the cavity.

Place the chicken on a rack in a roasting pan. Roast in the preheated oven for about 1 hour to 1 hour and 15 minutes, or until the internal temperature reaches 165°F (74°C) and the skin is golden brown and crispy. Baste occasionally with chicken broth if using.

Remove the chicken from the oven and let it rest for about 10-15 minutes before carving.

Spicy Chicken Lettuce Wraps

(per serving, 4 wraps):

Calories: 300

Fat: 18g

Protein: 25g

Carbs: 12g

Fiber: 3g

Sugars: 6g

Prep Time: 15 minutes Cooking Time: 10 minutes Total Time: 25 minutes
Serving Size: 4 wraps (about 1 cup of filling per wrap)

1 lb ground chicken

1 tablespoon olive oil

1 small onion, finely chopped

2 cloves garlic, minced

1 tablespoon fresh ginger, minced

1 red bell pepper, finely chopped

1 cup shredded carrots

2 tablespoons coconut aminos

1 tablespoon chili paste or hot sauce (adjust to taste)

1 teaspoon ground cumin

1 teaspoon paprika

Salt and pepper to taste

12 large lettuce leaves, iceberg or butter lettuce

1/4 cup chopped fresh cilantro

Lime wedges

In a large skillet, heat the olive oil over medium heat.

Add the onion, garlic, and ginger to the skillet. Sauté for about 3 minutes until fragrant and translucent.

Add the ground chicken to the skillet. Cook, breaking it up with a spoon, until browned and cooked through, about 5-7 minutes.

Stir in the red bell pepper and shredded carrots. Cook for an additional 2-3 minutes until vegetables are tender.

Add the coconut aminos, chili paste or hot sauce, ground cumin, paprika, salt, and pepper. Mix well and cook for another 2 minutes, allowing the flavors to combine.

Wash and dry the lettuce leaves. Arrange them on a serving platter.

Spoon the spicy chicken mixture into the center of each lettuce leaf.

Garnish with chopped cilantro and serve with lime wedges on the side, if desired.

Chicken and Sweet Potato Stew

((per serving, 1 cup):

Calories: 250

Fat: 10g

Protein: 23g

Carbohydrates: 24g

Fiber: 5g

Sugars: 6g

Prep Time: 15 minutes Cooking Time: 45 minutes Total Time: 1 hour
Serving Size: 1 cup (about 8 ounces)

1 lb (450g) boneless, skinless chicken thighs, cut into bite-sized pieces

2 medium sweet potatoes, peeled and diced

1 large carrot, peeled and sliced

1 onion, chopped

3 cloves garlic, minced

1 tablespoon olive oil

1 teaspoon ground turmeric

1 teaspoon ground cumin

1/2 teaspoon ground paprika

1/2 teaspoon dried thyme

1/2 teaspoon dried rosemary

4 cups low-sodium chicken broth

1 cup chopped kale or spinach (optional)

Salt and pepper to taste

Peel and dice the sweet potatoes and carrot. Chop the onion and mince the garlic.

In a large pot or Dutch oven, heat the olive oil over medium heat. Add the chopped onion and cook until translucent, about 5 minutes.

Add the chicken pieces and cook until lightly browned on all sides, about 5-7 minutes.

Stir in the minced garlic, turmeric, cumin, paprika, thyme, and rosemary. Cook for 1 minute until fragrant.

Add the diced sweet potatoes, sliced carrot, and chicken broth. Stir to combine.

Bring the stew to a boil, then reduce the heat to low. Cover and simmer for 30-35 minutes, or until the sweet potatoes and carrots are tender and the chicken is cooked through.

If using, stir in the chopped kale or spinach and cook for an additional 5 minutes until wilted.

Season with salt and pepper to taste. Serve warm.

Rosemary Garlic Lamb Chops

((per serving, 2 lamb chops):

Calories: 350

Fat: 24g

Protein: 30g

Carbs: 0g

Fiber: 0g

Sugars: 0g

Prep Time: 10 minutes Cooking Time: 15 minutes Total Time: 25 minutes
Serving Size: 2 lamb chops

4 lamb chops (about 1 inch thick)

2 tablespoons olive oil

3 cloves garlic, minced

2 tablespoons fresh rosemary, chopped
or 2 teaspoons dried rosemary

1 teaspoon salt

1/2 teaspoon black pepper

1/2 teaspoon lemon zest

In a small bowl, combine olive oil, minced garlic, rosemary, salt, pepper, and lemon zest (if using). Rub this mixture all over the lamb chops.

Allow the lamb chops to marinate for at least 10 minutes. For more intense flavor, you can marinate them for up to 1 hour in the refrigerator.

Heat a large skillet or grill pan over medium-high heat.

Add the lamb chops to the hot pan. Cook for about 4-5 minutes per side for medium-rare, or longer if desired.

Remove the lamb chops from the pan and let them rest for 5 minutes before serving.

Ginger-Turmeric Beef Stir-Fry

((per serving):

Calories: 350

Fat: 20g

Protein: 30g

Carbohydrates: 15g

Fiber: 4g

Sugars: 7g

Prep Time: 15 minutes Cooking Time: 10 minutes Total Time: 25 minutes
Serving Size: 1 cup (about 1 serving)

1 pound (450g) beef sirloin, thinly sliced

1 tablespoon coconut oil

1 tablespoon fresh ginger, minced

1 tablespoon fresh turmeric, minced or 1 teaspoon ground turmeric

2 cups bell peppers, sliced (red and yellow)

1 cup broccoli florets

1 medium carrot, sliced

1 tablespoon tamari (gluten-free soy sauce) or coconut aminos

1 tablespoon lime juice

1 tablespoon sesame seeds

Salt and pepper to taste

Slice the beef and vegetables. Mince the ginger and turmeric or use ground turmeric.

In a large skillet or wok, heat the coconut oil over medium-high heat.

Add the sliced beef to the skillet and stir-fry for about 3-4 minutes until browned and cooked through. Remove beef from the skillet and set aside.

In the same skillet, add the minced ginger and turmeric. Stir-fry for about 1 minute until fragrant.

Add the bell peppers, broccoli, and carrots to the skillet. Stir-fry for about 5 minutes until vegetables are tender-crisp.

Return the cooked beef to the skillet. Add tamari or coconut aminos and lime juice. Stir to combine and cook for an additional 2 minutes.

Season with salt and pepper to taste. Garnish with sesame seeds if desired.

Serve the stir-fry hot over steamed rice or cauliflower rice.

Spiced Turkey Meatballs

((per serving of 4 meatballs):

Calories: 240

Fat: 14g

Protein: 22g

Carbs: 6g

Fiber: 2g

Sugars: 1g

Prep Time: 15 minutes Cooking Time: 25 minutes Total Time: 40 minutes
Serving Size: 4 meatballs (about 1.5 inches in diameter)

1 lb ground turkey

1/2 cup finely chopped onion

2 cloves garlic, minced

1/4 cup fresh parsley, chopped

1/4 cup almond flour

1 large egg

1 teaspoon ground cumin

1/2 teaspoon ground paprika

1/2 teaspoon ground turmeric

1/4 teaspoon ground black pepper

1/4 teaspoon ground cinnamon

1/2 teaspoon salt

1 tablespoon olive oil

Preheat your oven to 400°F (200°C). Line a baking sheet with parchment paper or lightly grease it.

In a large bowl, combine the ground turkey, chopped onion, minced garlic, parsley, almond flour, egg, cumin, paprika, turmeric, black pepper, cinnamon, and salt. Mix until well combined but don't overmix.

Shape the mixture into meatballs, about 1.5 inches in diameter, and place them on the prepared baking sheet.

Drizzle the meatballs with olive oil. Bake for 20-25 minutes, or until the meatballs are cooked through and have an internal temperature of 165°F

(74°C).

Let the meatballs rest for a few minutes before serving.

Beef and Vegetable Kebabs

(per serving, 2 kebabs):

Calories: 350

Fat: 20g

Protein: 30g

Carbs: 15g

Fiber: 4g

Sugars: 8g

Prep Time: 15 minutes Cooking Time: 10-15 minutes Total Time: 1 hour 30 minutes Serving Size: 2 kebabs (1/2 pound of beef and vegetables)

1 pound beef sirloin or tenderloin, cut into 1-inch cubes

1 red bell pepper, cut into chunks

1 green bell pepper, cut into chunks

1 zucchini, sliced into rounds

1 red onion, cut into chunks

2 tablespoons olive oil

2 tablespoons balsamic vinegar

1 tablespoon lemon juice

2 cloves garlic, minced

1 teaspoon dried oregano

1 teaspoon dried thyme

1 teaspoon paprika

1/2 teaspoon ground black pepper

1/2 teaspoon salt

In a bowl, mix olive oil, balsamic vinegar, lemon juice, garlic, oregano, thyme, paprika, black pepper, and salt.

Add beef cubes to the marinade and toss to coat. Cover and refrigerate for at least 1 hour (or overnight for more flavor).

Preheat the grill or grill pan to medium-high heat.

Thread the marinated beef, bell peppers, zucchini, and onion onto skewers, alternating between beef and vegetables.

Grill the kebabs for 10-15 minutes, turning occasionally, until the beef is cooked to your desired level of doneness and vegetables are tender.

Remove from the grill and let rest for a few minutes before serving.

Turmeric-Spiced Shrimp

((per serving):

Calories: 150

Fat: 8g

Protein: 18g

Carbs: 2g

Fiber: 0g

Sugars: 0g

Prep Time: 10 minutes Cooking Time: 10 minutes Total Time: 20 minutes
Serving Size: 2 servings (about 4-6 shrimp per serving)

12 large shrimp, peeled and deveined

1 tablespoon olive oil

1 teaspoon ground turmeric

1/2 teaspoon ground cumin

1/2 teaspoon paprika

1/4 teaspoon ground black pepper

1/4 teaspoon garlic powder

1/4 teaspoon ground ginger

1/4 teaspoon salt (optional, to taste)

1 tablespoon lemon juice

Fresh cilantro or parsley

In a medium bowl, combine the olive oil, turmeric, cumin, paprika, black pepper, garlic powder, ginger, salt, and lemon juice. Add the shrimp and toss to coat evenly. Let it marinate for at least 10 minutes.

Heat a large skillet over medium heat.

Add the marinated shrimp to the hot skillet. Cook for 2-3 minutes on each side, or until the shrimp are opaque and cooked through.

Transfer the shrimp to a plate and garnish with fresh cilantro or parsley, if desired.

Mackerel with Tomato and Olive Relish

Prep Time: 10 minutes Cooking Time: 10 minutes Total Time: 20 minutes
Serving Size: 2 servings

(per serving):

Calories: 350

Fat: 25g

Protein: 25g

Carbs: 8g

Fiber: 3g

Sugars: 4g

For the Mackerel:

2 mackerel filets

1 tablespoon olive oil

Salt and pepper, to taste

1 lemon (cut in half, one half juiced, the other half cut into wedges for serving)

For the Tomato and Olive Relish:

1 cup cherry tomatoes, quartered

1/4 cup Kalamata olives, pitted and sliced

1 tablespoon capers, drained

1 small red onion, finely chopped

2 tablespoons fresh parsley, chopped

1 tablespoon extra-virgin olive oil

1 tablespoon balsamic vinegar

Salt and pepper, to taste

Prepare the Mackerel:

 - Season the mackerel filets with salt, pepper, and lemon juice.

 - Heat the olive oil in a large skillet over medium-high heat.

 - Add the mackerel filets, skin-side down, and cook for 3-4 minutes until the skin is crispy.

 - Flip the filets and cook for another 2-3 minutes until the fish is cooked through.

Make the Tomato and Olive Relish:

- In a medium bowl, combine the cherry tomatoes, olives, capers, red onion, parsley, olive oil, and balsamic vinegar.

- Season the relish with salt and pepper to taste and toss well.

Serve:

- Plate the mackerel filets and spoon the tomato and olive relish over the top.

- Serve with lemon wedges on the side.

Sardine Salad

((per serving):

Calories: 350

Fat: 28g

Protein: 18g

Carbs: 8g

Fiber: 5g

Sugars: 2g

Prep Time: 10 minutes Total Time: 10 minutes Serving Size: 1 salad

1 can (3.75 oz) sardines packed in olive oil, drained

1 cup mixed greens (arugula, spinach, or your choice)

1/4 cup cherry tomatoes, halved

1/4 cucumber, sliced

1/4 red onion, thinly sliced

1 tablespoon capers, drained

1 tablespoon fresh lemon juice

1 tablespoon extra-virgin olive oil

1/2 avocado, sliced

Salt and pepper to taste

Fresh herbs like parsley or dill

Place the mixed greens in a large bowl or on a plate.

Top the greens with cherry tomatoes, cucumber, red onion, and capers.

Gently place the sardines on top of the salad.

Drizzle the salad with lemon juice and olive oil. Season with salt and pepper to taste.

Arrange the avocado slices around the salad.

Garnish with fresh herbs if desired.

Tuna and White Bean Salad

((per serving):

Calories: 320

Fat: 14g

Protein: 27g

Carbs: 24g

Fiber: 8g

Sugars: 2g

Prep Time: 10 minutes Total Time: 10 minutes Serving Size: 2 servings

1 can (5 oz) tuna packed in water, drained

1 can (15 oz) white beans like cannellini or great northern, drained and rinsed

1/4 cup red onion, finely chopped

1/4 cup fresh parsley, chopped

2 tablespoons extra virgin olive oil

1 tablespoon lemon juice (freshly squeezed)

1 teaspoon Dijon mustard

Salt and pepper to taste

1/2 cup cherry tomatoes, halved; 1/4 cup cucumber, diced

Drain and rinse the white beans. Drain the tuna. Chop the red onion, parsley, and any optional vegetables you wish to add.

In a large bowl, combine the tuna, white beans, red onion, and parsley. Add the cherry tomatoes and cucumber if using.

In a small bowl, whisk together the olive oil, lemon juice, Dijon mustard, salt, and pepper.

Pour the dressing over the tuna and bean mixture. Toss gently until everything is well coated.

Divide the salad into two portions and serve or refrigerate for later.

Garlic-Lemon Scallops

(per serving):

Calories: 250

Fat: 14g

Protein: 25g

Carbs: 6g

Fiber: 1g

Sugars: 1g

Prep Time: 10 minutes Cooking Time: 10 minutes Total Time: 20 minutes
Serving Size: 2 servings

1 lb large sea scallops, cleaned and patted dry

2 tablespoons olive oil or avocado oil

3 garlic cloves, minced

Juice and zest of 1 lemon

1 tablespoon fresh parsley, chopped

Salt and pepper to taste

Lemon wedges for serving

Pat the scallops dry with a paper towel to ensure a good sear. Season both sides with salt and pepper.

Heat the olive oil in a large skillet over medium-high heat. Once the oil is hot, add the scallops in a single layer. Sear for about 2-3 minutes on each side until they develop a golden-brown crust. Remove the scallops from the pan and set aside.

In the same pan, reduce the heat to medium and add the minced garlic. Sauté for 1 minute, stirring constantly, until fragrant.

Add the lemon juice and zest to the pan, stirring to combine with the garlic.

Place the scallops back into the pan, tossing them in the garlic-lemon sauce. Cook for another minute to heat through.

Transfer the scallops to a serving plate, drizzle with any remaining sauce from the pan, and sprinkle with fresh parsley. Serve with lemon wedges on the side.

Herring with Beet Salad

(per serving):

Serving Size: 1 bowl about 1 1/2 cups

Calories**: 220

Protein**: 18g

Fat**: 4g

Carbs: 26g

Fiber: 4g

Calcium: 200 mg

Prep Time: 15 minutes Cooking Time: 30 minutes Total Time: 45 minutes
Serving Size: 1 plate (about 1 cup salad and 1 herring filet)

For the Salad:

2 medium beets, cooked and diced

1 small red onion, finely chopped

1 apple, diced (optional for sweetness)

1 tablespoon fresh dill, chopped

1 tablespoon apple cider vinegar

2 tablespoons olive oil

Salt and pepper to taste

For the Herring:

1-2 herring filets (pickled or smoked)

Lemon wedges

Fresh dill

If using raw beets, boil or roast them until tender, about 30 minutes. Let them cool, then peel and dice.

In a large bowl, combine the diced beets, chopped red onion, and diced apple (if using). Add the fresh dill, apple cider vinegar, and olive oil. Toss well to combine. Season with salt and pepper to taste.

Place the herring filets on a plate. Squeeze a little lemon juice over the top and garnish with fresh dill, if desired.

Plate the beet salad alongside the herring filets.

GRAINS AND LEGUMES

Brown Rice and Black Bean Burrito

(Calories per Serving: 350

Fat: 8g

Protein: 14g

Carbs: 60g

Prep Time: 10 minutes Cooking Time: 30 minutes Serving Size: 4 servings

For the Bowl:

1 cup brown rice

1 can (15 oz) black beans, drained and rinsed

1 cup corn kernels (fresh, frozen, or canned)

1 red bell pepper, diced

1 cup cherry tomatoes, halved

1 avocado, diced

1/4 cup chopped fresh cilantro

Juice of 1 lime

For the Dressing:

2 tablespoons extra-virgin olive oil

1 tablespoon apple cider vinegar

1 teaspoon ground cumin

1/2 teaspoon smoked paprika

1/2 teaspoon garlic powder

1/4 teaspoon ground turmeric

Salt and pepper to taste

Rinse the brown rice in cold water. In a medium pot, mix 1 cup of brown rice with 2 cups of water. Bring to a boil, then decrease the heat to low, cover, and simmer for approximately 30 minutes, or until the rice is cooked and the water is absorbed. Fluff with a fork and let it cool somewhat.

In a large bowl, mix the black beans, corn, sliced red bell pepper, cherry tomatoes, and chopped cilantro. Add the lime juice and stir to blend thoroughly.

In a small bowl, mix together the olive oil, apple cider vinegar, cumin, smoked paprika, garlic powder, turmeric, salt, and pepper.

Divide the cooked brown rice into 4 dishes. Top each bowl with the black bean and veggie mixture. Add chopped avocado on top of each bowl.

Drizzle the dressing over the bowls before serving.

Barley and Mushroom Risotto

(Calories per Serving: 280

Fat: 6g

Protein: 8g

Carbs: 45g

Prep Time: 10 minutes Cooking Time: 40 minutes Serving Size: 4 servings

1 cup pearled barley

2 tablespoons olive oil

1 medium onion, finely chopped

3 cloves garlic, minced

2 cups mushrooms, sliced, cremini or shiitake

1/2 cup dry white wine

4 cups vegetable broth

1 cup water (more as needed)

1/2 teaspoon dried thyme or 1 teaspoon fresh thyme

1/2 teaspoon dried rosemary or 1 teaspoon fresh rosemary

1/2 teaspoon turmeric

1/4 cup nutritional yeast

Salt and black pepper

Rinse the pearled barley under cold water and leave aside.

Heat olive oil in a large pan over medium heat. Add the chopped onion and simmer until transparent, approximately 5 minutes. Add the minced garlic and simmer for another 1-2 minutes until fragrant.

Add the sliced mushrooms to the pan and sauté until they are browned and soft, approximately 8-10 minutes.

Stir in the rinsed barley and simmer for 1-2 minutes. If using, pour in the white wine and simmer until it is largely absorbed.

Add 1 cup of vegetable broth and mix until it is largely absorbed. Continue adding the broth, one cup at a time, allowing it to be absorbed before adding the next cup. Stir regularly. You may also add water if the mixture gets too thick.

When the barley is soft and creamy (after around 30-40 minutes), toss in the thyme, rosemary, turmeric, and nutritional yeast if using. Season with salt and black pepper to taste.

Once the risotto has a creamy consistency, remove from heat and serve warm.

Red Lentil Curry

(Calories per Serving: 250

Fat: 8g

Protein: 13g

Carbs: 35g

Prep Time:10 minutes Cooking Time: 30 minutes Serving Size: 4 servings

1 cup red lentils, rinsed and drained	1 tablespoon curry powder
1 tablespoon coconut oil or olive oil	1 teaspoon ground turmeric
1 medium onion, chopped	1 teaspoon ground cumin
3 garlic cloves, minced	1/2 teaspoon paprika
1 tablespoon fresh ginger, minced	1/2 teaspoon ground coriander
1 can (14.5 oz) diced tomatoes	1/2 teaspoon black pepper
1 cup coconut milk (unsweetened)	1/2 teaspoon sea salt or to taste
2 cups vegetable broth (low sodium)	1 cup spinach

In a big saucepan, heat the coconut oil over medium heat. Add the chopped onion and simmer until transparent, approximately 5 minutes. Add the minced garlic and ginger, and simmer for another 1-2 minutes until fragrant.

Stir in the curry powder, turmeric, cumin, paprika, coriander, black pepper, and salt. Cook for around 1 minute to toast the seasonings.

Add the chopped tomatoes, coconut milk, and vegetable broth to the saucepan. Stir well to mix.

Add the washed red lentils. Bring the mixture to a boil, then decrease the heat to low and cover. Simmer for around 20-25 minutes, or until the lentils are soft and the curry has thickened. Stir periodically to avoid sticking.

If using, toss in the spinach until wilted. Adjust seasoning to taste if required. Serve hot over rice or with a side of naan.

Millet and Vegetable Stir-Fry

(Calories per Serving: 250

Fat: 7g

Protein: 8g

Carbs: 35g

Prep Time: 15 minutes Cooking Time: 20 minutes Serving Size: 4 servings

1 cup millet

2 cups water or vegetable broth

1 tablespoon olive oil (or avocado oil)

1 medium onion, diced

2 cloves garlic, minced

1 bell pepper, sliced

1 medium zucchini, sliced

1 cup broccoli florets

1 cup snap peas

1 medium carrot, julienned

2 tablespoons tamari (gluten-free soy sauce) or coconut aminos

1 tablespoon fresh ginger, grated

1/2 teaspoon ground turmeric

1/2 teaspoon ground black pepper

1 tablespoon sesame seeds

Fresh cilantro or green onions

Rinse the millet under cold water. In a medium saucepan, mix the millet and water or vegetable broth. Bring to a boil, then decrease heat to low, cover, and simmer for approximately 15 minutes, or until the liquid is absorbed and the millet is soft. Remove from heat and let it rest covered for 5 minutes, then fluff with a fork.

While the millet is cooking, heat the olive oil in a large pan or wok over medium-high heat. Add the diced onion and simmer for 3-4 minutes until softened.

Add the minced garlic and heat for a further minute. Then, add the bell pepper, zucchini, broccoli, snap peas, and carrot. Stir-fry the veggies for approximately 5-7 minutes, or until they are crisp-tender.

Add the tamari or coconut aminos, grated ginger, crushed turmeric, and black pepper to the veggies. Stir well to coat the veggies evenly with the spices.

Add the cooked millet to the pan with the veggies. Stir well to incorporate and cook through, approximately 2-3 minutes.

Garnish with sesame seeds and fresh cilantro or green onions if preferred. Serve warm.

For extra crunch, you may also add a handful of roasted nuts or seeds.

Chickpea and Spinach Curry

(Calories per Serving: 300

Fat: 10g

Protein: 12g

Carbs: 40g

Prep Time: 10 minutes Cooking Time: 20 minutes Serving Size: 4 servings

1 tablespoon olive oil

1 medium onion, finely chopped

3 garlic cloves, minced

1 tablespoon fresh ginger, minced

1 teaspoon ground turmeric

1 teaspoon ground cumin

1 teaspoon ground coriander

1/2 teaspoon paprika

1/2 teaspoon cayenne pepper

1 can (15 oz) chickpeas, drained and rinsed

1 can (14.5 oz) diced tomatoes (no added sugar)

1 cup vegetable broth

4 cups fresh spinach, washed and chopped

1/2 cup coconut milk (canned)

Salt and pepper

1 tablespoon fresh lemon juice

Heat olive oil in a large pan over medium heat. Add the chopped onion and simmer until transparent, approximately 5 minutes. Add the minced garlic and ginger, simmering for another 1-2 minutes until fragrant.

Stir in the ground turmeric, cumin, coriander, paprika, and cayenne pepper (if using). Cook for 1 minute to toast the seasonings.

Add the drained chickpeas, diced tomatoes, and vegetable broth. Stir to incorporate and bring to a simmer. Reduce heat and let it simmer for approximately 10 minutes to enable the flavors to mingle.

Stir in the chopped spinach and coconut milk. Cook for another 2-3 minutes until the spinach is wilted and the curry is cooked through.

Season with salt and pepper to taste. If preferred, add a tablespoon of fresh lemon juice for added taste. Serve hot over rice or with gluten-free naan.

Adjust Spice Levels: The cayenne pepper provides spice but may be eliminated if you want a milder curry.

Quinoa and Sweet Potato Chili

Calories per Serving: 300

Fat: 7g

Prep Time: 15 minutes Cooking Time: 35 minutes Serving Size: 4 servings

Protein: 11g

Carbs: 49g

1 tablespoon olive oil

1 large onion, diced

2 cloves garlic, minced

1 large bell pepper, diced

2 medium sweet potatoes, peeled and diced

1 cup quinoa, rinsed

1 can (14.5 oz) diced tomatoes (no salt added)

1 can (15 oz) black beans, drained and rinsed

1 can (15 oz) kidney beans, drained and rinsed

1 cup vegetable broth (low sodium)

1 tablespoon ground cumin

1 tablespoon smoked paprika

1 teaspoon ground turmeric

1/2 teaspoon ground chili powder

Salt and pepper

1 cup frozen corn

1/4 cup chopped fresh cilantro

Heat olive oil in a big saucepan over medium heat. Add the chopped onion and sauté until transparent, approximately 5 minutes. Add minced garlic and simmer for another 1-2 minutes until fragrant.

Stir in the chopped bell pepper and sweet potatoes. Cook for approximately 5 minutes, stirring periodically.

Add the rinsed quinoa, chopped tomatoes, black beans, kidney beans, vegetable broth, cumin, smoked paprika, turmeric, chili powder, salt, and pepper. Stir well to mix.

Bring the mixture to a boil, then decrease the heat to low. Cover and let it boil for 20-25 minutes, or until the sweet potatoes are soft and the quinoa is cooked. If using frozen corn, mix it in during the final 5 minutes of cooking.

Taste the chili and adjust seasoning if required. Garnish with fresh cilantro if desired.

Ladle the chili into bowls and serve hot.

Wild Rice and Cranberry Salad

(Calories per Serving: 220

Fat: 7g

Protein: 6g

Carbs: 32g

Prep Time: 15 minutes Cooking Time: 35 minutes Serving Size: 4 servings

1 cup wild rice	2 tablespoons olive oil
2 1/2 cups water or vegetable broth	1 tablespoon apple cider vinegar
1/2 cup dried cranberries	1 tablespoon fresh lemon juice
1/4 cup chopped walnuts (or pecans)	1 teaspoon Dijon mustard
1/4 cup finely chopped red onion	1/2 teaspoon dried thyme
1/2 cup diced celery	Salt and pepper
1/2 cup diced apple	

Rinse the wild rice under cold water. In a medium saucepan, bring 2 1/2 cups water or vegetable broth to a boil. Add the wild rice, lower heat to low, cover, and simmer for approximately 35 minutes, or until the rice is soft but chewy. Drain any extra liquid and allow the rice cool to room temperature.

While the rice is cooking, cut the red onion, celery, and apple (if using). Toast the walnuts in a dry pan over medium heat for 5 minutes or until aromatic, then let them cool.

In a small bowl, mix together the olive oil, apple cider vinegar, lemon juice, Dijon mustard, dried thyme, salt, and pepper.

In a large bowl, mix the cooked wild rice, dried cranberries, chopped walnuts, red onion, celery, and apple. Pour the dressing over the salad and toss to coat evenly.

Let the salad rest in the refrigerator for at least 30 minutes to enable the flavors to mingle. Toss again before serving.

Black Bean and Corn Salad

Calories per Serving: 220

Fat: 6g

Protein: 8g

Carbs: 33g

Prep Time: 15 minutes Serving Size: 4 servings

1 can (15 oz) black beans, drained and rinsed

1 cup fresh or frozen corn kernels (if frozen, thawed)

1 red bell pepper, diced

1 cup cherry tomatoes, halved

1/4 cup red onion, finely chopped

1/4 cup fresh cilantro, chopped

1 avocado, diced

2 tablespoons extra-virgin olive oil

Juice of 1 lime

1/2 teaspoon ground cumin

1/2 teaspoon smoked paprika

Salt and pepper

Drain and rinse the black beans. If using frozen corn, defrost it by putting it in a basin of water or running it under cold water.

In a large bowl, add the black beans, corn, diced red bell pepper, cherry tomatoes, red onion, and chopped cilantro.

In a small bowl, mix together the olive oil, lime juice, ground cumin, smoked paprika, salt, and pepper.

Pour the dressing over the salad and toss lightly to mix. Add the diced avocado and mix gently to prevent mashing the avocado.

Let the salad rest for approximately 10 minutes to enable the flavors to mingle. Serve refrigerated or at room temperature.

Bulgur Wheat and Chickpea Salad

Calories per Serving: 250

Fat: 7g

Protein: 9g

Carbs: 36g

Prep Time: 15 minutes Cooking Time: 10 minutes Serving Size: 4 servings

1 cup bulgur wheat

1 1/2 cups water or vegetable broth

1 can (15 oz) chickpeas, drained and rinsed

1 cup cherry tomatoes, halved

1 cucumber, diced

1/4 cup red onion, finely chopped

1/4 cup fresh parsley, chopped

1/4 cup fresh mint, chopped

1/4 cup extra virgin olive oil

Juice of 1 lemon

1/2 teaspoon ground turmeric

1/2 teaspoon ground cumin

Salt and pepper

In a medium saucepan, bring 1 1/2 cups of water or vegetable broth to a boil. Add the bulgur wheat, decrease heat to low, cover, and simmer for 10 minutes until the liquid is absorbed and the bulgur is soft. Remove from heat and allow it to cool to room temperature.

While the bulgur is cooking, cut the cherry tomatoes, cucumber, red onion, parsley, and mint.

In a large bowl, mix the cooked bulgur wheat, chickpeas, cherry tomatoes, cucumber, red onion, parsley, and mint.

In a small bowl, mix together the olive oil, lemon juice, turmeric, cumin, salt, and pepper.

Pour the dressing over the salad and mix until all ingredients are well-coated.

Adjust seasoning with extra salt and pepper if required.

Let the salad rest for at least 15 minutes to enable flavors to blend. Serve refrigerated or at room temperature.

Bulgur Wheat includes gluten, thus this dish is not ideal for persons with food intolerance. You may replace quinoa or rice for a gluten-free alternative.

Quinoa and Black Bean Tacos

(Calories per Serving: 350

Fat: 8g

Protein: 14g

Carbs: 55g

Prep Time: 15 minutes Cooking Time: 20 minutes Serving Size: 4 tacos

For the Quinoa and Black Bean Filling:

1 cup quinoa, rinsed

2 cups water

1 can (15 oz) black beans, drained and rinsed

1 tablespoon olive oil

1 small onion, diced

2 cloves garlic, minced

1 red bell pepper, diced

1 cup corn kernels (fresh, frozen, or canned)

1 teaspoon ground cumin

1/2 teaspoon smoked paprika

1/2 teaspoon chili powder

1/2 teaspoon turmeric

Salt and pepper

For Serving:

4 gluten-free taco shells or tortillas

1 avocado, sliced

1 cup shredded lettuce

1/2 cup cherry tomatoes, halved

Fresh cilantro leaves, chopped

Lime wedges

In a medium saucepan, bring 2 cups of water to a boil. Add the rinsed quinoa, lower heat to low, cover, and simmer for approximately 15 minutes, or until the quinoa is cooked and the water is absorbed. Fluff with a fork and put aside.

While the quinoa cooks, heat olive oil in a large pan over medium heat. Add the chopped onion and sauté until transparent, approximately 5 minutes. Add the minced garlic and simmer for another 1 minute.

Stir in the diced red bell pepper and simmer for 3 minutes. Add the corn, cooked quinoa, black beans, cumin, smoked paprika, chili powder, and turmeric. Cook for another 5-7 minutes, stirring periodically, until cooked through and thoroughly mixed. Season with salt and pepper to taste.

Warm the gluten-free taco shells or tortillas according to package directions. Divide the quinoa and black bean mixture equally among the taco shells.

Top each taco with sliced avocado, shredded lettuce, cherry tomatoes, and chopped cilantro, if using. Serve with lime wedges on the side.

SOUPS AND STEWS

Turmeric Chicken Soup

(per serving):

Calories: 300

Fat: 20g

Protein: 20g

Carbs: 15g

Fiber: 4g

Sugars: 5g

Prep Time: 15 minutes Cooking Time: 30 minutes Total Time: 45 minutes
Serving Size: 1 bowl (about 2 cups) Servings: 4

1 lb (about 450g) boneless, skinless chicken thighs or breasts, cut into bite-sized pieces

1 tablespoon olive oil

1 large onion, diced

3 cloves garlic, minced

1 tablespoon fresh ginger, grated

1 tablespoon ground turmeric

1 teaspoon ground cumin

1 teaspoon ground coriander

4 cups chicken broth (gluten-free)

1 can (14 oz) coconut milk (optional for a creamier soup)

2 large carrots, sliced

2 celery stalks, sliced

1 zucchini, diced

1 cup baby spinach

Juice of 1 lemon

Salt and pepper, to taste

Fresh cilantro or parsley, for garnish

In a large pot, heat the olive oil over medium heat. Add the diced onion and sauté until softened, about 5 minutes. Add the garlic and ginger, and sauté for another minute until fragrant.

Add the chicken pieces to the pot and cook until browned on all sides, about 5-7 minutes.

Stir in the turmeric, cumin, and coriander, cooking for another minute to release the spices' aromas.

Pour in the chicken broth and coconut milk (if using). Add the carrots, celery, and zucchini. Bring the soup to a boil, then reduce the heat and let it simmer for 20 minutes, until the vegetables are tender and the chicken is cooked through.

Stir in the baby spinach and lemon juice, and season with salt and pepper to taste. Cook for another 2-3 minutes, until the spinach is wilted.

Ladle the soup into bowls and garnish with fresh cilantro or parsley. Serve warm

Miso Soup with Tofu

(per serving):

Calories: 90

Fat: 3g

Protein: 7g

Carbs: 8g

Fiber: 2g

Sugars: 1g

Prep Time: 10 minutes Cooking Time: 10 minutes Total Time: 20 minutes
Serving Size: 1 bowl (about 12 ounces)

4 cups water or vegetable broth

3 tablespoons miso paste

1/2 cup firm tofu, cubed

1/2 cup chopped green onions (scallions)

1/2 cup sliced shiitake mushrooms

1/4 cup wakame seaweed, rehydrated

1 tablespoon tamari or gluten-free soy sauce

If using dried wakame seaweed, soak it in water for 5 minutes until rehydrated, then drain and set aside.

In a medium-sized pot, bring the water or vegetable broth to a gentle simmer over medium heat.

Add the tofu, green onions, shiitake mushrooms, and rehydrated wakame seaweed to the pot. Simmer for about 5 minutes until the mushrooms are tender and the tofu is heated through.

Reduce the heat to low. Place the miso paste in a small bowl, add a ladle of hot broth, and whisk until smooth. Add the diluted miso back into the soup and stir well. Do not boil the soup after adding the miso, as this can destroy its beneficial probiotics.

Add tamari or gluten-free soy sauce if desired for extra flavor. Adjust to taste.

Ladle the soup into bowls and serve warm.

Quinoa Vegetable Soup

(per serving):

Calories: 210

Fat: 5g

Protein: 7g

Carbs: 35g

Fiber: 7g

Sugars: 7g

Prep Time: 10 minutes Cooking Time: 25 minutes Total Time: 35 minutes
Serving Size: 1 bowl (about 1 1/2 cups)

1/2 cup quinoa, rinsed

1 tablespoon olive oil

1 onion, diced

2 carrots, diced

2 celery stalks, diced

3 garlic cloves, minced

1 zucchini, diced

1 red bell pepper, diced

1 can (14.5 ounces) diced tomatoes

6 cups vegetable broth

1 teaspoon ground turmeric

1 teaspoon ground cumin

1/2 teaspoon ground coriander

1/2 teaspoon smoked paprika

1/2 teaspoon dried thyme

Salt and pepper to taste

2 cups kale or spinach, chopped

1/4 cup fresh parsley, chopped
(for garnish)

1 tablespoon lemon juice

In a medium saucepan, bring 1 cup of water to a boil. Add the quinoa, reduce the heat to low, cover, and simmer for about 15 minutes until the quinoa is cooked and the water is absorbed. Set aside.

In a large pot, heat the olive oil over medium heat. Add the onion, carrots, celery, and garlic. Sauté for 5-7 minutes until the vegetables are softened.

Stir in the zucchini, red bell pepper, and diced tomatoes. Cook for another 3 minutes.

Add the turmeric, cumin, coriander, smoked paprika, thyme, salt, and pepper.

Pour in the vegetable broth, stir well, and bring the soup to a boil.

Reduce the heat and let the soup simmer for 15 minutes.

Stir in the cooked quinoa and chopped kale or spinach. Simmer for another 5 minutes until the greens are wilted.

Stir in the lemon juice if using. Ladle the soup into bowls, garnish with fresh parsley, and serve warm.

Cabbage and Kale Soup

((per serving):

Calories: 120

Fat: 4g

Protein: 4g

Carbs: 18g

Fiber: 6g

Sugars: 8g

Prep Time: 10 minutes Cooking Time: 30 minutes Total Time: 40 minutes
Serving Size: 1 bowl (about 2 cups)

1 tablespoon olive oil

1 medium onion, diced

2 garlic cloves, minced

4 cups green cabbage, chopped

2 cups kale, chopped (stems removed)

2 carrots, sliced

1 celery stalk, sliced

1 can (14.5 oz) diced tomatoes (no salt added)

6 cups vegetable broth (low-sodium)

1 teaspoon turmeric

1/2 teaspoon ground cumin

1/2 teaspoon ground black pepper

1/2 teaspoon paprika

Salt to taste (optional)

Juice of 1/2 lemon

Heat the olive oil in a large pot over medium heat. Add the diced onion and garlic, and sauté until the onion becomes translucent, about 5 minutes.

Stir in the chopped cabbage, kale, carrots, and celery. Cook for another 5 minutes, stirring occasionally.

Add the diced tomatoes, vegetable broth, turmeric, cumin, black pepper, and paprika. Stir well to combine.

Bring the soup to a boil, then reduce the heat to low and let it simmer for 20-25 minutes, or until the vegetables are tender.

Taste and adjust the seasoning with salt if needed. Stir in the lemon juice if using, and serve the soup hot.

Turkish Red Lentil Soup

((per serving):

Calories: 180

Fat: 4g

Protein: 9g

Carbs: 28g

Fiber: 7g

Sugars: 4g

Prep Time: 10 minutes Cooking Time: 30 minutes Total Time: 40 minutes
Serving Size: 1 bowl (about 1 1/2 cups) Servings: 4

1 cup red lentils, rinsed

1 medium onion, finely chopped

1 carrot, peeled and diced

2 cloves garlic, minced

1 tablespoon olive oil

1 tablespoon tomato paste

1 teaspoon ground cumin

1/2 teaspoon ground paprika or smoked paprika

1/4 teaspoon ground turmeric

1/4 teaspoon ground black pepper

4 cups vegetable broth (or water)

1 teaspoon salt (or to taste)

1 lemon, cut into wedges (for serving)

Fresh parsley, chopped

In a large pot, heat the olive oil over medium heat. Add the chopped onion, carrot, and garlic. Sauté for 5 minutes, or until the onion becomes translucent and the vegetables are softened.

Stir in the tomato paste, cumin, paprika, turmeric, and black pepper. Cook for an additional 2 minutes, allowing the spices to become fragrant.

Add the rinsed red lentils and vegetable broth (or water) to the pot. Stir to combine.

Bring the mixture to a boil, then reduce the heat to low. Cover and let it simmer for about 20-25 minutes, or until the lentils are soft and the soup has thickened.

For a smoother texture, use an immersion blender to blend the soup until creamy. You can also leave it chunky if you prefer.

Taste and adjust the seasoning with salt if necessary.

Ladle the soup into bowls and serve with lemon wedges for squeezing over the top. Garnish with fresh parsley if desired.

Mushroom Barley Soup

(per serving):

Calories: 250

Fat: 5g

Protein: 7g

Carbs: 45g

Fiber: 8g

Sugars: 4g

Prep Time: 15 minutes Cooking Time: 45 minutes Total Time: 1 hour
Serving Size: 1 bowl (about 1 1/2 cups)

1 tablespoon olive oil	1 cup pearl barley
1 medium onion, diced	6 cups vegetable broth
2 cloves garlic, minced	1 teaspoon dried thyme
2 carrots, diced	1 bay leaf
2 celery stalks, diced	Salt and pepper to taste
8 ounces mushrooms, sliced, cremini or button mushrooms work well	1 tablespoon fresh parsley, chopped

Heat olive oil in a large pot over medium heat. Add the onion, garlic, carrots, and celery. Sauté for about 5 minutes until the vegetables begin to soften.

Add the sliced mushrooms to the pot and cook for another 5 minutes until they release their moisture and begin to brown.

Stir in the pearl barley, vegetable broth, dried thyme, and bay leaf. Bring the mixture to a boil.

Reduce the heat to low, cover, and simmer for about 45 minutes, or until the barley is tender and the soup has thickened. Stir occasionally.

Remove the bay leaf, then season the soup with salt and pepper to taste.

Ladle the soup into bowls and garnish with fresh parsley if desired. Serve hot.

Spicy Chickpea Soup

(per serving):

Calories: 250

Fat: 6g

Protein: 8g

Carbohydrates: 40g

Fiber: 10g

Sugars: 8g

Prep Time: 10 minutes Cooking Time: 30 minutes Total Time: 40 minutes
Serving Size: 1 bowl (about 1.5 cups)

1 tablespoon olive oil

1 small onion, diced

2 cloves garlic, minced

1 teaspoon ground cumin

1 teaspoon ground coriander

1/2 teaspoon ground turmeric

1/4 teaspoon cayenne pepper (adjust to taste)

1/4 teaspoon smoked paprika

1 can (15 ounces) chickpeas, drained and rinsed

1 can (14.5 ounces) diced tomatoes

4 cups vegetable broth

1 small sweet potato, peeled and diced

1/2 teaspoon sea salt (adjust to taste)

1/4 teaspoon black pepper

1 cup chopped spinach or kale

Juice of 1/2 lemon

Fresh cilantro

In a large pot, heat the olive oil over medium heat. Add the diced onion and cook until translucent, about 5 minutes. Add the minced garlic and cook for another minute

Stir in the ground cumin, coriander, turmeric, cayenne pepper, and smoked paprika. Cook for 1-2 minutes until fragrant.

Add the chickpeas and diced tomatoes to the pot. Stir well to coat them with the spices.

Pour in the vegetable broth and add the diced sweet potato. Bring the soup to a boil, then reduce the heat and let it simmer for about 20-25 minutes, or until the sweet potato is tender.

Stir in the chopped spinach or kale, if using, and let it wilt into the soup for about 2-3 minutes.

Season the soup with salt and black pepper to taste. Serve hot, with a squeeze of fresh lemon juice and a sprinkle of cilantro, if desired.

Cauliflower and Leek Soup

(per serving):

Calories: 120

Fat: 5g

Protein: 4g

Carbs: 16g

Fiber: 5g

Sugars: 4g

Prep Time: 10 minutes Cooking Time: 30 minutes Total Time: 40 minutes
Serving Size: 1 cup (about 8 ounces) Servings: 4

1 medium head of cauliflower, chopped into florets

2 large leeks, white and light green parts only, sliced

3 cloves garlic, minced

4 cups vegetable broth

1 tablespoon olive oil

1 teaspoon ground turmeric

1/2 teaspoon ground cumin

1/4 teaspoon ground black pepper

Salt to taste

Fresh parsley or chives

Wash and chop the cauliflower into small florets. Slice the leeks and rinse them thoroughly to remove any grit.

In a large pot, heat the olive oil over medium heat. Add the sliced leeks and garlic, and sauté until the leeks are soft, about 5 minutes.

Add the cauliflower florets to the pot along with the turmeric, cumin, black pepper, and a pinch of salt. Stir to coat the vegetables with the spices.

Pour in the vegetable broth and bring the mixture to a boil. Reduce the heat to low, cover the pot, and let it simmer for about 20 minutes, or until the cauliflower is tender.

Use an immersion blender to blend the soup until smooth and creamy. Alternatively, you can carefully transfer the soup in batches to a blender and blend until smooth.

Taste and adjust the seasoning with more salt if needed.

Ladle the soup into bowls and garnish with fresh parsley or chives if desired.

Pumpkin and Coconut Milk Soup

((per serving):

Calories: 200

Fat: 16g

Protein: 2g

Carbs: 15g

Fiber: 3g

Sugars: 6g

Prep Time: 10 minutes Cooking Time: 30 minutes Total Time: 40 minutes
Serving Size: 1 bowl (about 1 cup)

1 tablespoon coconut oil

1 small onion, diced

2 cloves garlic, minced

1 teaspoon fresh ginger, grated

1 teaspoon ground turmeric

1/2 teaspoon ground cumin

1/4 teaspoon ground cinnamon

4 cups pumpkin puree or 1 small pumpkin, peeled, seeded, and cubed

3 cups vegetable broth

1 can (14 ounces) full-fat coconut milk

Salt and pepper to taste

1 tablespoon fresh lime juice

Fresh cilantro

In a large pot, heat the coconut oil over medium heat. Add the diced onion and sauté until soft and translucent, about 5 minutes. Add the garlic, ginger, turmeric, cumin, and cinnamon, and cook for another minute until fragrant.

Stir in the pumpkin puree or cubed pumpkin, and cook for 2-3 minutes, allowing the flavors to blend.

Pour in the vegetable broth, bring to a boil, then reduce the heat and let it simmer for about 20 minutes, or until the pumpkin is tender (if using cubed pumpkin).

Using an immersion blender, blend the soup until smooth. Alternatively, transfer the soup to a blender and blend in batches, then return it to the pot.

Stir in the coconut milk and lime juice, and season with salt and pepper to taste. Simmer for another 5 minutes until the soup is heated through.

Ladle the soup into bowls and garnish with fresh cilantro, if desired. Serve warm.

PART 4: LIFESTYLE PRACTICES FOR REDUCING INFLAMMATION

Stress and Inflammation: Breaking the Cycle

Stress and inflammation are inextricably intertwined, forming a cycle that may be difficult to interrupt. When you're stressed, your body produces stress chemicals such as cortisol and adrenaline. These chemicals prepare your body to adapt to acute dangers, but prolonged stress may cause long-term inflammation. Understanding this relationship is critical for successful stress and inflammation management.

Chronic stress may have a significant influence on your health, causing persistent inflammation. Here's what happens:

- Stress Hormones: When you are stressed, your body secretes cortisol and adrenaline. Although these hormones are necessary for short-term reactions, extended exposure may disrupt your immune system and promote inflammation
- Immune System Dysregulation: Chronic stress can induce an overactive immune system, resulting in an excessive inflammatory response. This may cause tissue damage and contribute to several inflammatory diseases.
- Gut Health: Stress may disrupt the gut microbiota, causing an imbalance in bacteria. This imbalance may cause inflammation in the gut and throughout the body
- Behavioral Factors: Stress can lead to unhealthy habits including poor nutrition, lack of exercise, and insufficient sleep, which can contribute to inflammation.

Natural Techniques for Stress Reduction: Breathing, Meditation, and Grounding

Managing stress is critical for lowering inflammation and improving overall health. Here are some natural ways that might help:

1. Breathing Exercises:
- Deep Breathing: Deep breathing may stimulate the parasympathetic nervous system, leading to relaxation and reduced stress. Try breathing deeply through your nose, holding your breath for a few seconds before gently exhaling through your mouth.

- Box Breathing: This method consists of breathing for four seconds, holding the breath for four seconds, expelling for four seconds, then holding the breath again for four seconds. Repeat the cycle numerous times to relax your mind and body.

2. Meditation:
- Mindfulness Meditation: Focus on the now and observe thoughts and emotions without judgment. Regular mindfulness meditation may help decrease stress and inflammation.
- Guided Meditation: Using guided meditation recordings may help you relax and decrease stress. These recordings often feature soothing music and instructions to help you concentrate and relax.

3. Grounding (Earthing):
- Walking barefoot: Grounding includes barefoot contact with the ground, such as walking on grass, sand, or dirt. This exercise may help decrease stress and inflammation by instilling a feeling of connectedness to nature.
- Grounding Mats: If going barefoot outdoors isn't an option, grounding mats may provide comparable advantages. These mats are intended to simulate an electrical connection with the ground and may be used inside.

Exercise: Moving for Healing

Exercise is an effective method for lowering inflammation and improving overall health. Regular physical exercise helps to regulate the immune system, enhance circulation, and reduce stress, all of which lead to decreased inflammation. Incorporating exercise into your regular routine will dramatically improve your health and help your body recover naturally.

Not all exercise must be strenuous to be successful. Gentle exercises may also alleviate inflammation and give a variety of health advantages. Here are some moderate exercises that are quite useful:

1. Walking: Walking is a basic and easily accessible method of exercise. It improves circulation, reduces stress, and promotes cardiovascular health. Even a 20-minute stroll might have anti-inflammatory benefits. Begin with short walks, gradually increasing the time and intensity. Aim to walk for at least 30 minutes most days of the week.

2. Stretching benefits include maintaining flexibility, improving range of motion, and reducing muscular tension. It may also increase blood flow to the muscles, which helps with recuperation and reduces inflammation. Include stretching in your everyday regimen. Concentrate on main muscle groups, holding each stretch for at least 30 seconds. Avoid jumping and stretch slowly to prevent injury.

3. Yoga: Yoga promotes relaxation and reduces stress via physical postures, breathing exercises, and meditation. It enhances flexibility, strength, and balance while lowering inflammation. Begin with beginner-level yoga courses or online lessons. Beginners and those trying to lessen inflammation might benefit from gentle yoga styles like Hatha or Yin.

The Benefits of Stretching, Yoga, and Walking

Stretching, yoga, and walking may all help reduce inflammation and improve overall health. Here's how each of these activities promotes healing:

1. Stretching:
- Flexibility and Mobility: Regular stretching promotes muscular flexibility and joint health, lowering the risk of injury and increasing mobility.
- Stress Relief: Stretching may relieve muscular tension, promote relaxation, and reduce stress, resulting in decreased inflammation.

2. Yoga:
- Mind-Body Connection: Yoga helps improve awareness and reduce stress. This comprehensive method manages inflammation and promotes general well-being.
- Physical Benefits: Yoga enhances strength, flexibility, and balance, promoting overall health and lowering inflammation.

3. Walking:
- Cardiovascular Health: Walking enhances cardiovascular health, lowering inflammation and promoting general health.
- Mental Health: Walking outside may improve mood, decrease anxiety, and increase mental clarity, all of which lead to lower inflammation level.

Sleep: The Forgotten Healer

Sleep is sometimes disregarded when it comes to sustaining health and lowering inflammation, despite its importance in both. Quality sleep helps the body to repair and rejuvenate, which improves immunological function and lowers the risk of chronic illnesses. Understanding the value of sleep and how to enhance it may have a big influence on your overall well-being.

Poor sleep may cause inflammation in a variety of ways:

- Stress Hormones: Sleep deprivation increases cortisol levels, which can cause inflammation in the body
- Immune System Dysregulation: Sleep deprivation disrupts the immune system's balance, leading to overproduction of pro-inflammatory cytokines

- Blood Vessel Health: Sleep reduces blood pressure and relaxes blood vessels. Insufficient sleep may hinder relaxation, possibly triggering inflammatory cells in blood vessel walls
- Glymphatic System: The brain's waste-clearing system is most active during deep sleep. Inadequate sleep disrupts this mechanism, causing inflammatory proteins to accumulate.

Chronic sleep deprivation may lead to inflammatory illnesses including heart disease, diabetes, and Alzheimer's disease.

Establishing a Sleep Sanctuary for Healing

Creating an atmosphere favorable to peaceful sleep is critical for lowering inflammation and encouraging recovery. Here are some suggestions to help you build a sleep sanctuary:

1. Invest in comfortable bedding, including a mattress and pillows that provide enough support. The appropriate bedding may dramatically enhance sleep quality.
   - Bedding Materials: Use breathable, natural textiles like cotton or linen for sheets and blankets to maintain body warmth.

2. For an optimal sleep environment, keep your bedroom as dark as possible. To prevent light from disrupting melatonin synthesis, use blackout curtains or an eye mask.
   - Quiet: Reduce noise by using earplugs or utilizing a white noise machine. A calm setting improves sleep quality and duration.
   - Cool Temperature: Keep your bedroom cool, preferably between 60 and 67°F (15 and 19°C). A colder environment signals to the body that it's time for sleep.

3. Sleep Routine: Maintain a consistent schedule by going to bed and waking up at the same time every day, including weekends. Maintaining a regular sleep pattern helps maintain your body's internal clock.
   - A Relaxing Pre-Sleep Routine: Create a relaxing sleep ritual to indicate to your body that it's time to relax. This might include things like reading, taking a warm bath, or doing mild yoga.

4. Limit Stimulants: Avoid coffee and alcohol before bedtime. Both may interrupt sleep patterns and lower sleep quality.
   - Electronic Devices: Limit your screen time (phones, tablets, and TVs) before bedtime. These gadgets generate blue light, which may disrupt melatonin production.

5. Mindfulness and Relaxation:
   - Meditation and Breathing Exercises: Practicing mindfulness meditation or deep breathing exercises before bedtime may decrease stress and promote relaxation.

- Gratitude Journaling: Keeping a gratitude journal helps reduce stress and promote a pleasant sleep mindset.

PART 5: HOLISTIC HEALING APPROACHES

Sunshine and fresh air: Nature's Free Medicine

Spending time outside in the sun and fresh air is one of the most easy and effective strategies to improve your health. Nature provides several advantages that may improve both physical and mental well-being. Nature's healing potential is deep and available to everyone, ranging from mood enhancement to inflammation reduction.

Vitamin D, sometimes known as the "sunshine vitamin," is created by the body when exposed to sunlight. It is essential for general health and contains potent anti-inflammatory compounds. Here's how vitamin D may lower inflammation:

- Immune System Modulation: Vitamin D regulates the immune system, allowing it to respond correctly to threats without overreacting. This regulation helps avoid chronic inflammation, which may contribute to a number of health concerns.
- Reduction of Pro-Inflammatory Cytokines: Vitamin D inhibits the synthesis of pro-inflammatory cytokines, which cause inflammation. It also boosts the production of anti-inflammatory cytokines, which helps to regulate the immune system.
- Promotes Bone Health: Vitamin D levels are necessary for calcium absorption and bone health maintenance. Healthy bones are less likely to become inflamed or develop conditions like osteoporosis
- Protection against Autoimmune Diseases: Research suggests that vitamin D can help reduce the risk of autoimmune diseases, which occur when the immune system incorrectly attacks the body's own tissues, causing inflammation.

Spend time outside in the sun to obtain adequate vitamin D, particularly in the mornings and late afternoons when the sun is less powerful. Fatty fish, fortified dairy products, and egg yolks are all sources of vitamin D, and supplements may be taken as needed.

How Nature Helps the Body Heal

Nature has an amazing potential to help the body's healing processes. Here are several ways in which spending time outside might improve your health:

- Stress Reduction: Being in nature reduces stress levels by decreasing the synthesis of stress hormones such as cortisol. Lower stress levels are linked to better health and lower inflammation.
- Exposure to natural surroundings may also boost mood, reduce anxiety, and increase cognitive function. This emotional well-being leads to improved physical health and a stronger immune system.
- Improved Immune Function: Exposure to fresh air and sunshine helps strengthen the immune system, enhancing its ability to fight infections and reduce inflammation
- Physical Activity: Engaging in outdoor activities such as walking, hiking, and gardening promotes good weight management, cardiovascular health, and inflammation reduction.
- Connection with Nature: Nature promotes connection and well-being. This relationship may increase attention and relaxation, enhancing the body's healing processes.

To receive the advantages of nature, plan to spend at least two hours every week outside. This time may be stretched out over many days and may include activities such as strolling in the park, hiking, or just relaxing in a garden. The idea is to include frequent outside activities into your daily routine.

In conclusion, sunlight and fresh air are potent natural remedies that may dramatically improve your health. Spending time outside and getting enough vitamin D may help decrease inflammation, improve your immune system, and support your body's natural healing processes. Embrace nature's healing power and include it into your normal holistic health activities.

The Benefits of Detox Baths and Skin Care

Detox baths and natural skin care are effective ways to reduce inflammation and improve general health. Incorporating these activities into your daily routine will help your body's natural detoxification processes while also improving the health and look of your skin.

Epsom Salt Baths & Natural Skin Care for Inflammation

1. Epsom Salt Baths: Epsom salt (magnesium sulfate) may decrease inflammation, alleviate muscular tension, and promote relaxation. Epsom salts dissolve in warm water and may be absorbed via the skin, thereby increasing magnesium levels in the body. To make an Epsom salt bath, pour 2 cups of Epsom salts into a warm bath and soak for at least 20 minutes. This promotes magnesium absorption and detoxification via the skin.
- Additional Ingredients: Enhance your detox bath with essential oils such as lavender or eucalyptus for anti-inflammatory and soothing properties.

2. Natural Skin Care:

- Gentle Cleansing: Use natural, gentle cleansers that do not remove the skin's natural oils. Look for products that have calming and anti-inflammatory components such as aloe vera, chamomile, and green tea. Regular exfoliation removes dead skin cells and increases cell turnover, resulting in healthier and more vibrant skin. Natural exfoliants, such as sugar or oats, are gentle on the skin.
- Moisturizing: Natural moisturizers such as coconut oil, shea butter, and jojoba oil may help keep your skin moisturized. These compounds prevent moisture loss and defend against environmental stressors.

The Importance of Detoxifying via the Skin

Detoxifying via your skin is an excellent technique to help your body's detoxification processes. Here's why it matters:

- Biggest Organ: The skin is the body's biggest organ and plays an important function in toxin removal. Sweating helps the skin cleanse pollutants and regulate body temperature.
- Improved Circulation: Detox baths and skin care routines may boost blood circulation, delivering oxygen and nutrients to the skin and tissues. Detox baths and natural skin care may promote healthy skin and decrease inflammation by increasing circulation and eliminating toxins. This is especially good for disorders including eczema, psoriasis, and acne
- Enhanced Skin Health: Regular detoxification via the skin may result in cleaner, brighter, and younger-looking skin. It balances oil production, reduces blemishes, and improves skin texture.

MEAL PLANNING

Anti-Inflammatory Meal Plan: 30 Days to Healing

Week 1

Day 1
- Breakfast: Turmeric Latte
- Lunch: Beef and Vegetable Kebabs
- Dinner: Quinoa and Sweet Potato Chili

Day 2
- Breakfast: Berry-Kefir Smoothie
- Lunch: Vegan Buddha Bowl
- Dinner: Turmeric-Spiced Shrimp

Day 3
- Breakfast: Mango-Kale Smoothie
- Lunch: Chicken and Sweet Potato Stew
- Dinner: Vegan Lentil Soup

Day 4
- Breakfast: Cherry-Mocha Smoothie
- Lunch: Rosemary Garlic Lamb Chops
- Dinner: Turmeric Chicken Soup

Day 5
- Breakfast: Golden Milk
- Lunch: Sweet Potato-Black Bean Tacos
- Dinner: Ginger-Turmeric Beef Stir-Fry

Day 6
- Breakfast: Avocado-Banana Smoothie
- Lunch: Tuna and White Bean Salad
- Dinner: Chickpea and Spinach Curry

Day 7

- Breakfast: Beetroot Smoothie
- Lunch: Mackerel with Tomato and Olive Relish
- Dinner: Red Lentil Curry

Week 2

Day 8
- Breakfast: Pineapple-Ginger Smoothie
- Lunch: Caprese-Stuffed Portobello Mushrooms
- Dinner: Lentil and Spinach Stew

Day 9
- Breakfast: *Avocado & Kale Omelet
- Lunch: Sardine Salad
- Dinner: Mushroom Risotto

Day 10
- Breakfast: Blueberry-Spinach Smoothie
- Lunch: Quinoa and Black Bean Tacos
- Dinner: Spiced Turkey Meatballs

Day 11
- Breakfast: Spinach & Egg Scramble
- Lunch: Black Bean and Corn Salad
- Dinner: Turmeric Chicken

Day 12
- Breakfast: Egg Salad Avocado Toast
- Lunch: Brown Rice and Black Bean Burrito
- Dinner: Ginger-Garlic Chicken Stir-Fry

Day 13
- Breakfast: Turmeric Latte
- Lunch: Herring with Beet Salad
- Dinner: Vegetable Paella

Day 14
- Breakfast: Mango-Kale Smoothie
- Lunch: Tuna and White Bean Salad
- Dinner: Barley and Mushroom Risotto

Week 3

Day 15
- Breakfast: Cherry-Mocha Smoothie
- Lunch: Spicy Chicken Lettuce Wraps
- Dinner: Millet and Vegetable Stir-Fry

Day 16
- Breakfast: Golden Milk
- Lunch: Bulgur Wheat and Chickpea Salad
- Dinner: Pumpkin and Coconut Milk Soup

Day 17
- Breakfast: Avocado-Banana Smoothie
- Lunch: Quinoa Vegetable Soup
- Dinner: Lemon-Herb Roasted Chicken

Day 18
- Breakfast: Beetroot Smoothie
- Lunch: Wild Rice and Cranberry Salad
- Dinner: Cauliflower and Leek Soup

Day 19
- Breakfast: Blueberry-Spinach Smoothie
- Lunch: Mackerel with Tomato and Olive Relish
- Dinner: Ginger-Turmeric Beef Stir-Fry

Day 20
- Breakfast: Pineapple-Ginger Smoothie
- Lunch: Spiced Turkey Meatballs
- Dinner: Mushroom Barley Soup

Day 21
- Breakfast: Spinach & Egg Scramble
- Lunch: Vegan Buddha Bowl
- Dinner: Spicy Chickpea Soup

Week 4

Day 22

- Breakfast: Egg Salad Avocado Toast
- Lunch: Chickpea and Spinach Curry
- Dinner: Rosemary Garlic Lamb Chops

Day 23
- Breakfast: Turmeric Latte
- Lunch: Quinoa and Black Bean Tacos
- Dinner: Turkish Red Lentil Soup

Day 24
- Breakfast: Avocado & Kale Omelet
- Lunch: Herring with Beet Salad
- Dinner: Ginger-Garlic Chicken Stir-Fry

Day 25
- Breakfast: Berry-Kefir Smoothie
- Lunch: Caprese-Stuffed Portobello Mushrooms
- Dinner: Chickpea and Spinach Curry

Day 26
- Breakfast: Golden Milk
- Lunch: Sardine Salad
- Dinner: Vegetable Paella

Day 27
- Breakfast: Mango-Kale Smoothie
- Lunch: Black Bean and Corn Salad
- Dinner: Miso Soup with Tofu

Day 28
- Breakfast: Avocado-Banana Smoothie
- Lunch: Quinoa Vegetable Soup
- Dinner: Turmeric-Spiced Shrimp

Day 29
- Breakfast: Beetroot Smoothie
- Lunch: Brown Rice and Black Bean Burrito
- Dinner: Turmeric Chicken Soup

Day 30
- Breakfast: Blueberry-Spinach Smoothie
- Lunch: Lemon-Herb Roasted Chicken

- Dinner: Red Lentil Curry

Anti-Inflammatory Snacks and Treats (Store-Bought)

1. Nuts and Seeds
   - Almonds, walnuts, and chia seeds are rich in omega-3s and antioxidants. Look for raw or lightly salted options.
   - Brands like Blue Diamond or Navitas Organics offer organic nut mixes or chia seed pouches.

2. Dark Chocolate (70% or Higher)
   - High-quality dark chocolate with minimal sugar and at least 70% cacao has anti-inflammatory properties due to its high antioxidant content.
   - Look for brands like Lindt or Alter Eco.

3. Turmeric Chips
   - Many brands are now creating snacks with turmeric seasoning for an anti-inflammatory boost.
   - Bare Snacks offers turmeric-infused vegetable chips.

4. Pumpkin Seeds (Pepitas)
   - Pumpkin seeds are high in magnesium and antioxidants. Raw or roasted with sea salt makes for a perfect snack.
   - Brands like SuperSeedz or Terrasoul offer a variety of flavored options.

5. Hummus and Vegetable Sticks
   - Pre-packaged hummus cups paired with carrot or celery sticks are great anti-inflammatory options.
   - Brands like Sabra or Hope Foods offer small snack packs.

6. Greek Yogurt (Unsweetened)
   - Unsweetened, full-fat Greek yogurt provides probiotics and protein, which helps fight inflammation.
   - Brands like Fage or Chobani offer convenient single-serving options. Pair with anti-inflammatory toppings like berries or nuts.

7. Baked Seaweed Snacks
   - Seaweed is rich in antioxidants and omega-3s, which help reduce inflammation.
   - Brands like GimMe or SeaSnax offer baked seaweed snacks in various flavors.

8. Olives

- Olives are packed with anti-inflammatory oleic acid. Pre-packaged olives are great for quick snacking.
- Brands like Pearls or Mario Camacho have convenient pouches of olives.

9. Coconut Chips
- Coconut chips offer a crunchy, anti-inflammatory snack option. They are high in healthy fats and fiber.
- Dang and Bare offer lightly sweetened or plain coconut chips.

10. Dried Fruit (No Added Sugar)
- Look for anti-inflammatory fruits like dried blueberries, cherries, or cranberries without added sugar.
- Brands like Made In Nature or Natierra offer organic options.

11. Beet Chips
- Beets are high in antioxidants and fight inflammation. Beet chips offer a crunchy, healthy alternative to regular potato chips.
- Rhythm Superfoods offers beet chips in various flavors.

12. Pre-Packaged Guacamole Cups
- Avocados are a great source of healthy fats that reduce inflammation. Pre-packaged guacamole cups paired with vegetable chips or raw veggies make an easy snack.
- Brands like Wholly Guacamole offer individual cups.

13. Lentil Chips
- Lentil-based chips are high in fiber and plant-based protein, making them an excellent anti-inflammatory snack.
- Harvest Snaps offers a variety of lentil-based crisps.

14. Protein Bars (Low Sugar)
- Look for bars with anti-inflammatory ingredients like turmeric, ginger, or omega-3-rich seeds and nuts.
- Brands like RXBAR or Kind offer bars made with whole ingredients and no artificial sugars.

15. Chia Seed Pudding Cups
- Chia seeds are rich in omega-3s and fiber. Some brands offer chia seed puddings pre-made and ready to go.
- Mamma Chia or Chia Co offer on-the-go chia pudding snacks.

16. Edamame
- Pre-packaged edamame (young soybeans) is rich in fiber, protein, and anti-inflammatory omega-3s.

- Look for frozen or ready-to-eat options from brands like Seapoint Farms.

17. Veggie Straws or Chips
   - Vegetable-based straws or chips made from sweet potatoes, carrots, or kale are good anti-inflammatory alternatives to regular chips.
   - Brands like Good Health or Simply 7 offer a variety of vegetable-based snacks.

18. Collagen Protein Snacks
   - Collagen-rich snacks help reduce inflammation and support joint health.
   - Vital Proteins offers collagen bars and bites in various flavors.

19. Frozen Dark Chocolate-Covered Berries
   - Frozen berries coated in dark chocolate are high in antioxidants and make a delicious anti-inflammatory treat.
   - Brookside offers dark chocolate-covered blueberries and other berries.

20. Sardine or Mackerel Pouches
   - Sardines and mackerel are rich in omega-3s and are perfect for a quick snack.
   - Brands like Wild Planet or King Oscar offer convenient, flavored pouches.

FLARE UP TRACKER

TEMPLATE

DATE: 1/10/24 – 30/10/24	
FOODS ELIMINATED	**FLARE UP SYMPTOMS**

DATE: 1/11/24 – 7/11/24	
FOODS REINTRODUCED	**OBSERVATIONS**

| | |
| | |

| | |
| | |

Made in the USA
Las Vegas, NV
04 October 2024